succeeding

as a

hospital
doctor

the experts share
their secrets

Third edition

Roger Kirby and Tony Mundy

HEALTH PRESS

Succeeding as a Hospital Doctor
First published 2000
Second edition 2002
Third edition 2007

©2007 in this edition Health Press Limited
Health Press Limited, Elizabeth House, Queen Street, Abingdon, Oxford OX14 3LN, UK
Tel: +44 (0)1235 523233
Fax: +44 (0)1235 523238 www.healthpress.co.uk

A CIP catalogue record for this title is available from the British Library.

ISBN 978-1-903734-79-7

Kirby, R (Roger)
Succeeding as a Hospital Doctor/
Roger Kirby, Tony Mundy

Typesetting and page layout by Zed, Oxford, UK
Printed by Fine Print (Services) Ltd, Oxford, UK

Contents

Foreword

Success varies from person to person – and as this excellent volume demonstrates, often from text to picture; looking at the photographs we can see clearly that success comes in a variety of different physical forms. The common thread is optimism – all the contributors create confidence that the future of medicine is secure. That sense of 'can do' was not only important in their own development but is essential if improvements in health and healthcare are to be maintained in the years ahead.

This is a book to be enjoyed. The contrast between the formal chapters and the brief histories puts recent changes to the education, training and management of doctors in context. Of course we need accurate, up-to-date information on careers, research, communications, relationships with patients and colleagues and all the other factors that contribute to good medical practice and to a satisfying career. The surprise, however, is not how much has changed but rather how little the basic principles have altered over the years. Hippocrates wrote:

First of all I would define medicine as the complete removal of the distress of the sick, the alleviation of the more violent diseases and the refusal to undertake to cure cases in which the disease has already won the mastery, knowing that everything is not possible in medicine.

Not a bad definition, and one that has stood the test of time. Our first and overriding duty is still to care for and about our patients.

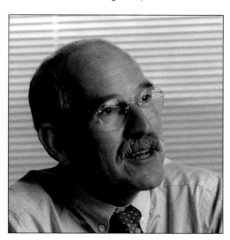

Of course the practical aspects of medical practice continue to change and improve. This book provides invaluable information on the many aspects of medicine that are seldom formally taught but are essential for a successful career – how to organize your time, your office and your practice. Patients and colleagues rightly expect us to have organizational as well as professional skills – always remembering that the science will change, society's expectations will change but people don't change. They will trust doctors when most burdened by ill-health and worries. That need for trust and humanity in medicine is unchanging. As this book makes abundantly clear, we must all in our different ways make patient care our first concern.

And yet, we can only do that if our personal lives outwith medicine are also balanced. As Hilaire Belloc put it

From quiet homes and first beginning
Out to the undiscovered ends,
There's nothing worth the wear of winning
But laughter and the love of friends.

Coming from the President of the GMC, that's optimism for you...

Professor Sir Graeme Catto
President, General Medical Council

Preface to the third edition

The idea for this book arose when we were asked to run a weekend course in Dublin entitled *Succeeding in Urology*. The meeting proved an ongoing success, so we set out to write a book, enlisted other experts to talk about their fields, and expanded our remit to cover other disciplines.

Since the first edition, we have seen the high-profile Bristol baby and Alder Hey pathology scandals provide the stimulus for the NHS Plan, calls for revalidation based on annual appraisal, and the negotiations over the new consultant contract. In the preface to the second edition, written as a result of these planned changes, we predicted stormy seas ahead for hospital medicine. We did not, however, anticipate the veritable tornado of change that has buffeted the profession since 2002. New Labour's reforming zeal has focussed on the health service and schools, because politicians know all too well that it is health and education that count in elections. A great deal of the unprecedented increase in funding has gone in increased salaries for doctors, which were welcome, but in return managers are turning the screw on doctors in an attempt to improve productivity. Financial pressures are beginning to bite as trusts struggle to balance their books, making redundancies of hospital doctors a distinct possibility. The strategic move of resources from secondary to primary care in order to 'treat patients closer to home' only compounds these pressures. Add to this the proposed changes in regulating the profession, the ongoing upheaval in training and the introduction of consumer power through 'patient choice' initiatives such as 'choose and book', and the need for a third edition of this book becomes obvious.

With this in mind, we have extensively updated and rewritten the text, and added a good deal of new material, including excellent new chapters from Alan Crockard, John Kelly and Michael Devlin. We have also invited some outstanding new 'voices of experience' to tell you how they did it and how it was for them, and we would like to thank all of our eminent contributors who have kindly shared their thoughts about the nature of success and how one may achieve it.

Despite the updating and changes in content, our principal aspirations for this book remain the same: we hope that the third edition will inspire many dedicated doctors to pilot their way successfully through the increasingly turbulent waters of a lifelong career in hospital medicine.

Roger Kirby and Tony Mundy

About the authors

Roger Kirby trained at Cambridge University and the Middlesex Hospital, London, and is visiting Professor of Urology at St George's Hospital, London and University College London. He is also Director of The Prostate Centre in London and Chairman and Secretary, respectively, of the Prostate Research Campaign UK and the British Urological Foundation, two fast-growing medical charities. Past Honorary Secretary of the British 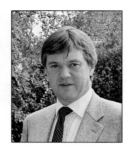 Association of Urological Surgeons, he launched and is Editor of the journal *Prostate Cancer and Prostatic Diseases* and associate editor of the *BJU International.* He is a prolific writer (this is his 56th book). Roger lives with his wife and three children in Wimbledon.

After qualifying from St Mary's Hospital Medical School, London, **Tony Mundy** trained in general surgery and then urology at Guy's Hospital. He is Professor of Urology at the University of London and Director of the Institute of Urology at University College London. He is Medical Director at University College London Hospitals NHS Foundation Trust, Member of Council of the Royal College of Surgeons of England and President of the British Association of Urological Surgeons.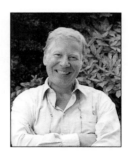

Chapter contributors

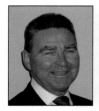 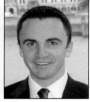 *Alan Crockard and Stuart Carney*
Training for success

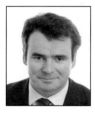 *John Kelly*
Research

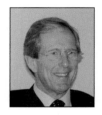 *Keith Parsons*
Management

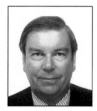 *Andrew Lang*
Finance

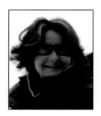 *Linky Trott*
Hiring and firing

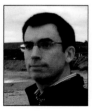 *Michael Devlin*
Medicolegal matters

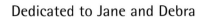

Dedicated to Jane and Debra

Introduction

What is a successful hospital career? The names of many eminent doctors may spring readily to mind – indeed, several have contributed to this volume – but defining the nature and means of their success is rather more difficult. In business, a high earning capacity is considered to be the hallmark of success, and there are literally hundreds of books telling you how to achieve it. Success in medicine, however, is considerably more subtle. Perhaps the best definition of a successful doctor is one who has gained a good reputation and credibility from the approval and respect of patients and colleagues alike (Table 1).

But how does one achieve such recognition and respect? First and foremost, be consistently ethical and professional in everything you do, remembering the words of Hippocrates, 'First do no harm'. Add to this three important principles:

- provide a high standard of practice and care
- maintain genuine relationships of trust with patients and colleagues
- be kind, honest and trustworthy in all aspects of professional practice.

Table 1
Successful people

- Set and achieve realistic goals
- Organize their time: free time; focus time; and buffer time enabling better focus time
- Invest in themselves by training
- Understand key relationships
- Have a passion for everything
- Are well supported by friends and family
- Show balance, honesty and integrity
- Are professional in everything that they do

Never forget the importance of making a meaningful connection with patients and colleagues. Add to this a focussed training, some fruitful research, well-honed communication skills and a good position in the NHS. A consistent track record is essential, as are effective management, communication, appraisal and team-building skills. Most importantly, learn to anticipate and avoid the pitfalls that lie in wait for us all, and if you do succumb, admit, face up to – and learn from – your mistakes, as well as from those of others.

So what are the benefits of success? If others perceive you as successful, this will help you as a clinician, researcher, manager and teacher. Remember, it is your reputation that goes before you and your image that is retained – and you are only as good as your last performance. Being considered a success will make the sometimes difficult task of dealing effectively with patients, colleagues and managers a great deal easier because of their preconceptions. It will also help you to build and sustain a solid team, as others become keen to join the bandwagon of your success, which will enable you to maintain a high and positive profile.

In this book, the building blocks and formulae for success are analysed, practical ways to achieve it are suggested, and advice on how to side-step the many potential pitfalls is provided. Although this book encompasses the views of some of the UK's leading doctors, it is not intended simply for the select few who aspire to the presidency of a Royal College or chairmanship of an august medical institution. Rather, it contains something for every trainee and qualified doctor. Each of us has the potential to be a little more successful than we actually are. We hope that this book will help many doctors achieve the happiness and sense of fulfilment that accompany a successful medical career.

training for success

Professor H Alan Crockard DSc FRCS(Eng) FRCP(Lond) FDS RCS(Eng)
Past National Director, Modernising Medical Careers (England)
and Dr Stuart Carney MPH MRCPsych
Specialist Registrar in Psychiatry, Oxford, and
Foundation School Director, Leicestershire, Northamptonshire
and Rutland Healthcare Workforce Deanery

'I am all for progress, it is change I object to'
Mark Twain (1835–1910)

On 1st August 2005, postgraduate medical training in the UK changed completely, shifting from an apprenticeship to a competence-based model. Why? Things surely were fine before that – or were they?

Increased patient expectations, the need to improve patient safety and the statutory reduction of the number of hours that doctors in training may work are having a profound impact on clinical services. Postgraduate medical education and training has had to evolve to meet these challenges. The new training pathways anticipate a health service in which the majority of front-line patient care is delivered by trained doctors working in clinical teams.

> this is **not a time** for **despair** for those who are **alive** to **change**

In this chapter we will explain why postgraduate training is changing and what it will look like. This is not a time for despair; rather, like all periods of revolution, it bears unrivalled and unexpected opportunities for those who are alive to change.

Background

Patient safety

By the end of the 1990s the medical profession had been rocked by not one but three high-profile scandals. Professor Ian Kennedy's investigation into the deaths of 29 babies undergoing heart surgery at the Bristol Royal Infirmary (see page 117) challenged the view that doctors know best and called for an end to the closed 'old boys' network'. The inquiry highlighted the need for greater involvement of patients in decisions about their treatment and care; the introduction of regular appraisal, continuing professional development and revalidation for doctors; and more openness about clinical performance.

The need for greater transparency and accountability of the medical profession were also among the conclusions of the Redfern report into the retention of children's body parts without their parents' consent at Alder Hey. However, perhaps the name that will be remembered above all others is that of the late Dr Harold Shipman, Britain's worst serial killer.

The last few years have also seen a series of audits and reviews, which have drawn attention to the large number of medical errors. On the surgical front, the National Confidential Enquiry into Perioperative Deaths (*Changing the way we operate* (2001)) revealed that the main contributory factors associated with perioperative deaths were junior doctors performing surgery, unsupervised and out of hours. For single conditions such as large bowel cancer or heart disease, mortality and morbidity varied hugely across the country. The best results were often in the busiest specialist units. The days of the occasional or infrequent operator are passing, as is the concept that every specialist in any district general hospital is equally skilled and successful.

> 'See one, do one, teach one' is no longer acceptable

It will not come as a surprise that education and training has come under the spotlight. 'See one, do one, teach one' is no longer acceptable. Instead doctors in training are expected to record or log all of their training experience and present evidence of their skills. Lessons learned from the aviation industry emphasize the value of breaking down procedures into their component parts, of simulation and of training as part of a team. The nuclear industry has demonstrated the importance of disaster planning and the need for checks to ensure safe practice. These have had a profound impact on training and practice, especially in emergency care. Advanced Life Support (ALS) training is just one example.

Service need

For decades hospitals have relied on doctors in training to provide most of the front-line medical care. In the middle of the night, care was typically provided by doctors in training, many of whom were on shifts of 24 hours or longer.

The focus on employees' health and safety and, more recently, patient safety has resulted in the extension of the requirements of the European Working Time Directive (EWTD) to doctors in training. This law, originally introduced to regulate the long hours of low-paid workers, will probably more profoundly affect the way medicine is delivered and how doctors are taught than any specific plans developed by the profession. Put simply, the 'firm' and apprenticeship model of training and delivery will not cope with the restrictions on working hours.

In addition, as pressures on trusts to deliver budgetary balance increase, and with the creation of foundation trusts, it is likely that traditional models for service delivery will be challenged in pursuit of better value, that is, clinical excellence will be scrutinized in the same equation as cost-effectiveness.

'Hospital at night', 'Hospital at weekend' and 'Hospital 24/7' are recent examples of a radical rethink of service delivery. These programmes have come into existence to keep people alive, and doctors are increasingly working a shift-pattern and providing cover for absent colleagues.

Patient choice

Patients no longer accept unquestioningly what the hospital doctor says; they can recognize good treatment and good doctors, particularly if they are supplied with enough information, and plenty of information is available on the internet. Patient choice is alive and rapidly expanding.

Many traditionally viewed hospital specialties are moving 'closer to home', into the community, to be more responsive to and convenient for patients. This shift in practice will require a completely different specialist and consultant workforce. For the first time some hospital consultants may only have a very tenuous attachment to their parent hospital.

Medical demography

In response to the need to increase the number of trained specialists, to comply with the requirements of the EWTD and to reduce reliance on medical graduates from abroad, the last decade has seen a 70% increase in the number of medical students. Women now make up 70% of the medical school class, and for the first time in the UK, there will be more female than male medical graduates in 2008.

change in disease management has **never** been **faster**

The attitudes of both male and female graduates have changed. They wish to excel in their chosen profession, but many have a significant life outside medicine. In attitude they are closer to the airline pilot than the one-track specialist of their predecessors. Training and service provision will have to change to accommodate this.

Changes in disease management

The pace of change in disease management has never been faster. The introduction of statins and stents over a 7-year period revolutionized the management of coronary heart disease, but it typically takes 12 years to train a heart surgeon. Endoscopes and radiological scanning have transformed urological and gynaecological disease management. There has been an 80% reduction in surgical interventions for some urological diseases, which suggests that fewer urologists should be trained to operate.

Who knows what impact stem cell research and gene manipulation will have on the practice of medicine? Whatever emerges, it is clear that greater flexibility is needed in the medical workforce, and training and trainees will need to be more responsive to changing service needs. It is likely that consultants just beginning their career will change their treatment methodologies or even their specialty every 10 to 15 years.

The 'lost tribe' and the structure of training

In 2002, the Chief Medical Officer published the consultation paper *Unfinished Business*. The report drew attention to the 'lost tribe' of Senior House Officers (SHOs), many of whom had spent years of unproductive time in the grade before securing a place in a specialty training programme. Although training was excellent in many areas, it was not consistent.

There were serious issues with many training programmes; they were not well planned, and doctors were variably supervised and increasingly expected to deliver heavy service workloads while in training. Government policy and intent to reform medical education was crystallized in the publication *Modernising Medical Careers: The Next Steps* in April 2004, which broadly defined the future shape of foundation, specialist and general practice training.

Raising standards

With the spotlight on the medical profession and the need to ensure independent and clear lines of accountability, regulation of postgraduate medical education passed by Act of Parliament to the Postgraduate Medical Education and Training Board (PMETB).

Established in September 2004, PMETB is responsible for setting the standards for postregistration medical education in the UK and making sure they are met. It is an independent statutory body and is answerable to Parliament. PMETB replaced the Specialist Training Authority (STA) and the Joint Committee for Postgraduate Training in General Practice (JCPTGP), which were essentially offshoots of the medical royal colleges. While royal colleges continue to develop curricula and assessment programmes, they must now conform to the explicit standards set by PMETB.

The role of the General Medical Council (GMC) in regulating undergraduate medical education and the first year of postgraduate training is under review (*Good Doctors, Safer Patients* (2006)). This is still work in progress and the ultimate shape of GMC/PMETB is not yet decided, but it is likely that throughout our working lives there will be much more explicit evaluation of our competences. We await the result of the consultation.

MMC and the new shape of postgraduate training

The evidence for the necessity of root-and-branch reform of postgraduate medical education was compelling.

When they established PMETB to raise standards, the four UK health ministers also set in train structural reforms under the banner 'Modernising Medical Careers' (MMC). The new MMC career structure and training programmes have been designed to give doctors a clear career path in which advancement is attained through the acquisition of explicit competences rather than time spent in a particular role. These changes should improve patient safety by ensuring junior doctors in their early years of training are well supervised and assessed against explicit standards, which are set out in the curricula for each specialty.

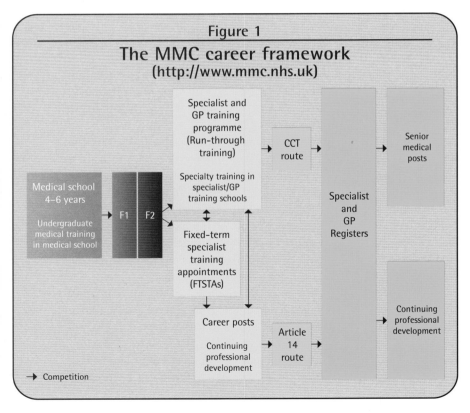

Figure 1

The MMC career framework (http://www.mmc.nhs.uk)

August 2005 saw the introduction of the foundation programme and 2007 the new unified specialist training or 'run-through' programme. The new shape of postgraduate training is shown in Figure 1.

From now on, medical graduates will train within managed training programmes according to an explicit curriculum. To succeed and progress you must gather evidence in your portfolio of your level of competence. This process of collecting evidence about your abilities should begin in medical school and is likely to continue throughout your medical career.

PMETB has defined clear principles for entry to specialist training. These principles have resulted in the development of national standards for recruitment, with transparent processes for the selection of all candidates applying for training places. The overall process of recruitment has been modernized by using an electronic portal to receive applications for foundation and specialist training, ultimately making it more efficient.

The goal of postgraduate training is entry onto the Specialist Register; PMETB sets the standards for entry. There are two routes for hospital doctors: Certificate of Completion of Training (CCT) or Certificate confirming Eligibility for the Specialist Register (CESR, otherwise known as the Article 14 equivalence route).

The foundation programme

In this section we describe the component parts of postgraduate training and give some tips on how to prepare for and make the most of training.

What is it?

Foundation training bridges the gap between medical school and specialist training. Organized around foundation schools, foundation programmes provide generic training for 2 years, including, where possible, a placement in primary care. Most schools also offer academic training opportunities, either integrated throughout the 2 years or just in the second year.

In the current regulatory framework, the GMC is responsible for the first year of foundation training (F1) and PMETB is responsible for the second year (F2). F1 equates to the old preregistration house officer year and is in fact the final year of basic medical education. For this reason, only those medical students who have to undertake a preregistration or equivalent internship year are eligible to apply. The competences for the foundation programme are described in the *Curriculum for the foundation years in postgraduate education and training* (2005). Successful completion of F1 results in full registration with the GMC, and after F2 a certificate of satisfactory completion is awarded. The principles, structures and requirements for foundation programmes are set out in the *Operational framework for foundation training* (2005).

The 2-year foundation programme seeks to enable you to:

- consolidate your knowledge, understanding and skills, and demonstrate that you meet nationally agreed levels of competence before you progress into specialist training
- reflect on your aspirations, abilities and service needs as you prepare for selection for specialist training.

Applying for foundation training

Medical students in the UK are required to undertake a preregistration year of training. This is not the case in all parts of Europe or the rest of the world. Only medical students who are required to undertake a preregistration year (or internship) are eligible to apply for 2-year foundation programmes (F1 and F2); there are places available for direct entry into F2 for other students.

There is a single online application process for 2-year foundation programmes (see the website of the Medical Training Application Service, http://www.mtas.nhs.uk). Your application is scored according to nationally agreed criteria by a panel. The overall score currently comprises an academic score provided by your medical school and the actual application score. The means by which medical schools provide an academic score is under review.

As with all applications, make sure you read the questions meticulously and keep to the prescribed word limit. The questions are mapped onto the requirements of the GMC's *Good Medical Practice* (2006) and relate to your ability to develop and maintain your medical knowledge and skills, work effectively as a member of a team and reflect on your practice. Examples can be drawn from your clinical training and experiences outside of medicine. This type of application process is totally different from anything before 2005; thus, informal discussions with those even a few years ahead will not provide you with a competitive edge.

Foundation training and gathering evidence of competence

The *Curriculum for the foundation years in postgraduate medical education and training* describes the knowledge, understanding and attitudes expected of foundation doctors. It is a 'spiral curriculum'; that is, competences such as history-taking and prescribing are visited in both years, with progressive development of skills and behaviours. The curriculum is designed to help you develop the competences necessary for ensuring patient safety and in particular the safe recognition, assessment and management of acutely ill patients.

During the foundation programme you must gather evidence in your portfolio that you have met the required standards of competence. There are a variety of assessment tools currently in use; they are intended to record your clinical competence from different perspectives in different clinical situations at an earlier stage in your training.

It is useful to reflect on why you are being assessed. Firstly, you are accountable to the public. Patients need assurance that you have demonstrated your ability to practise in accordance with the required standards. You need to show that

gather evidence that you have **met** the required **standards**

your overall performance is satisfactory before your foundation school director can recommend you to the GMC for full registration and subsequently certify that you have satisfactorily completed foundation year 2.

Secondly, assessment and feedback go hand in hand. Your personal development depends on constructive feedback. Choosing a career in medicine means you have chosen a career where you can look forward to lifelong learning and assessment. The goal of assessment is to help you provide better care and, if areas of weakness are identified, to help you improve accordingly.

During F1 you will be assessed against the standard of competence that is expected of a doctor completing the F1 year. This means that, in your first days as a foundation doctor, you are unlikely to reach the standard required. The assessments are designed to measure your progress through the year. At the end of F1, you will be expected to have progressed to a satisfactory level. Similarly during F2 you will be assessed against the standard of competence expected of a doctor completing the F2 year.

Foundation assessments are workplace-based – your educational supervisor will want to see what you actually do on the job and your ability to translate what you have learned into practice. Three types of assessment are commonly used.

- Multi-source feedback – this provides an opportunity for several of your colleagues to rate your abilities and offer comments. There are a number of tools currently in use, such as mini-ePAT, TAB and the Scottish multisource feedback tool. All require you to submit a list of colleagues as possible assessors. An administrator will contact the assessors and compile the results once sufficient responses are received. The report is sent to your educational supervisor, who will discuss the results and comments with you.
- Direct observation of doctor–patient interactions: the two most commonly used tools are Direct Observation of Procedural Skills (DOPS) and the Mini Clinical Evaluation Exercise (Mini-CEX). During your placements, you should ask experienced colleagues to observe you performing particular procedures (DOPS) or clinical consultations (mini-CEX), rate your level of competence and provide feedback. It is your responsibility to arrange the assessments and submit copies of the reports.
- Case-Based Discussion (CBD) – this is a structured review of cases you have been involved in. It allows you to discuss your decision-making and clinical reasoning.

You are responsible for organizing your own assessments. The assessments typically take no more than an hour each month. You must identify suitable cases and ask experienced colleagues to assess you. Do not leave your assessments until your final placement – your colleagues will not have time to complete all of the assessments in the last few weeks of F1 or F2!

Your educational supervisor will need to review your portfolio at regular intervals during F1 and F2. The assessments inform your educational supervisor's report to the foundation school at the end of F1 and F2. This is important to ensure you are recommended for full GMC registration at the end of F1 and for completion of the Foundation Achievement of Competency Document at the end of F2.

Bear in mind that 6 months into F2 you will enter the selection process for specialty training, so you should be thinking about what you want to do and how to fulfil the selection requirements (described in the next section) throughout your foundation years.

Specialty (run-through) training

Preparation

Selection into specialty training begins halfway through the second foundation year. Therefore you only have eighteen months after graduation to narrow your career options. You will have access to careers advice through your clinical or educational supervisor, as well as the careers management service in your foundation school or deanery.

You should review the person specifications of the specialties that interest you as you consider what direction you want your career to take. Specialty programme directors will be available to answer questions about individual specialties.

Competition can be tough. Many deaneries collect data about competition ratios. In 2005, the West Midlands Deanery received 12 applications for each old-style specialist registrar post in general surgery, 13 for each post in cardiology but only 2 for each child and adolescent psychiatry post. London, Kent, Surrey and Sussex and Eastern Deaneries received

> ## competition
> ### can be tough

17 applications for each post in general surgery, 6 for cardiology and 2 for child and adolescent psychiatry. Following national recruitment to new-style specialty registrar (StR) posts, these data should be more widely available. You should think widely and flexibly about your career options – consider a Plan A, B, C and possibly even D!

Applications for specialty training are made online according to a national timetable. Make sure that you check the application timetable and that you are available in case you are invited to interview. You must have a working e-mail address; invitations to interview and offers of appointment will be made by e-mail. Details about the national online application process can be found at http://www.mtas.nhs.uk.

In your application form you need to demonstrate that you have the skills and aptitude to begin a period of training in that particular speciality. If you are applying for entry at the ST1 (first-year) level, you are not expected to demonstrate that you have already acquired some training in that specialty, so a period in that particular speciality in the Foundation Programme is not an essential prerequisite for applying.

It is important to begin the process of gathering evidence early on in your foundation training. In addition to your clinical placements, tasters provide a useful opportunity to explore different career options. At a structured interview lasting at least 30 minutes, you will be expected to bring your portfolio to confirm that you are on target to complete foundation training and to corroborate what you have said in your application form.

tasters provide an **opportunity** to explore **options**

You must also identify two referees with whom you have worked clinically within the last 2 years. Most importantly, they will have to provide their references online within a very narrow time frame. You must make sure that your referees are aware of the timetable.

The specialty training programme

A new unified training programme replaces the old-style basic and advanced specialty training. These curriculum-driven 'run-through' programmes take you from from year 1 (ST1) through to the end of the training programme and entry onto the Specialist Register. As discussed above, there are two routes for entry onto the Specialist Register: Certificate of Completion of Training (CCT) and Certificate confirming Eligibility for Specialist Registration (CESR). CCT replaces the old Certificate of Satisfactory Completion of Training (CCST) and only applies if you have satisfactorily completed an entire course of specialty training. Irrespective of the route, once you are on the Specialist Register you can apply for a senior medical appointment.

Doctors entering specialty training from August 2007 will be called 'specialty registrars' (StRs). Subject to satisfactory progress, StRs will train in programmes that take them all the way through to the award of CCT. The predicted length of training ('indicative training length') will depend on the specialty. There are 58 specialties with training programmes leading to the award of a CCT. Some programmes include a common stem (e.g. Core Medical Training) based on old-style SHO training. The core phase of training will typically last 2 years, except in psychiatry, where it will last 3 years. Some specialty training programmes do not include a core training period (e.g. histopathology).

Figure 2 shows the shape of medical training. If you are interested in training in one of the 28 physician specialties (e.g. general internal medicine (acute), cardiology, gastroenterology), there are two pathways at ST1, namely, Core Medical Training and Acute Care Common Stem. Both programmes last 2 years and enable StRs to acquire and demonstrate level 1 competences in general internal medicine (acute). For StRs in these training programmes, there will be a competitive allocation process during ST2 for the physician specialties, for example from core medical training (CMT) into respiratory medicine.

The training pathways in surgery are shown in Figure 3. If you wish to become a neurosurgeon, you can apply for the neurosurgery run-through programme. Dually qualified doctors and dentists can apply for Oral and Maxillofacial Surgery. If you are interested in one of the other seven

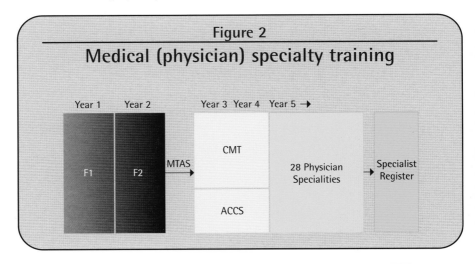

Figure 2
Medical (physician) specialty training

Year 1 Year 2 Year 3 Year 4 Year 5 →

F1 F2 MTAS → CMT / ACCS → 28 Physician Specialities → Specialist Register

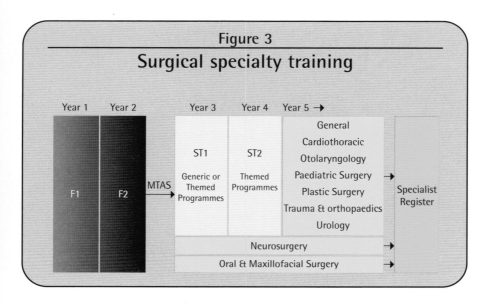

Figure 3

Surgical specialty training

surgical specialties, you should apply for either a themed or generic core surgical training programme. Surgical StRs in themed programmes will continue into the relevant surgical specialty subject to satisfactory progress; surgical StRs in generic programmes will compete for allocation to specialty.

The ACCS (Figure 4) includes placements in anaesthetics, critical care, emergency medicine and acute medicine. It leads on to training in the

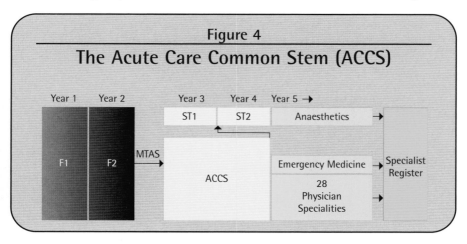

Figure 4

The Acute Care Common Stem (ACCS)

Training for success

28 physician specialties, emergency medicine and anaesthetics. Each of these three specialties/specialty groups will select separately for the themed ACCS programmes. ACCS is the only entry route for emergency medicine. Anaesthetics StRs recruited through ACCS will join the anaesthetics training programme at ST2. If you are interested in emergency medicine, acute medicine or combining intensive care medicine with either anaesthetics or medicine, then ACCS is right for you.

During core training in psychiatry there will also be an allocation/competition from the broad (core) programme into specific specialty programmes.

Like foundation training, your specialist training will be a managed programme following an approved curriculum with explicit way-points. You will be required to gather evidence of your knowledge, skills and level of competence. There will be regular review meetings. Details about the different specialty training programmes are available from the royal college websites (see the Further reading section at the end of this chapter).

Training abroad

Training episodes such as exchange programmes will require *prospective* approval from PMETB. PMETB will also review training obtained elsewhere; it may be considered equivalent to the training obtained in a UK training programme. However, without prior approval your training will not count towards a CCT, and entry to the Specialist Register will be via Article 14 equivalence route (CESR). While experience outside the

> **experience outside the UK** is still **encouraged**

UK is still encouraged, it is essential that you confirm with PMETB before you go that what you want to do abroad will be approved.

Fixed-term specialty training appointments

Many specialties or specialty groups offer fixed-term specialty training appointments (FTSTAs). These are 1-year appointments and provide the same training as the first, second or third year (psychiatry and paediatrics) of the appropriate run-through programme. However, they do not form part of a progressive training programme. Most doctors are likely to apply for a place in a specialty training programme, but you may prefer to apply for a FTSTA to consider alternative specialty careers. FTSTAs also provide the necessary training for work in a non-consultant career-grade post (NCCG); that is, you need a minimum of 2 years of relevant postfoundation specialty training to apply for career-grade posts in most specialties.

Appointment to a FTSTA carries no entitlement for entry into a run-through training programme in that specialty. The only way you can enter a run-through programme is through competitive appointment to the specialty training programme.

During the early part of transition, it is likely that FTSTA posts will be used to a greater extent to offer employment to those doctors who have already met the educational objectives of FTSTA year 1 and year 2 (and year 3 in psychiatry and paediatrics). Under such circumstances, you could use this opportunity to acquire additional experience and/or additional skills and competences which will be formally assessed, recorded and documented in your learning portfolio. If you are successful in gaining a place in a run-through programme in a relevant specialty, these achievements may be taken into account.

Applying for specialty training

Although it was originally planned that applications for specialty training would be made online to a common national timetable, a number of deficiencies in the novel computerized online application system (MTAS) and shortlisting process have become apparent. In particular, the validity of the application form for shortlisting has been called into question. At the time of writing a review group is working on improvements to the selection process. It is unclear how future recruitment rounds will be conducted, but whatever system is employed, applicants will be required to draw attention to their clinical skills, commitment to a given specialty, and academic and non-academic achievements. Suggestions about how to achieve success in these important areas are to be found elsewhere in this book. The latest information about the MTAS system is available from http://www.mtas.nhs.uk.

Training once you are on the Specialist Register

To succeed as a doctor you must be committed to lifelong learning. Dramatic developments in technology and other innovations have revolutionized medical practice. Training programmes cannot always keep pace with these changes. As we have already discussed, advances in the fields of urology and cardiac surgery have changed the shape of clinical practice, requiring fewer doctors to be competent in certain surgical procedures. Training in some procedures might only be given once you are on the Specialist Register. Trusts are responsible for determining the types of services and skills they need and will have to continue to train their workforce.

Academic training

Research is an essential part of the culture of medicine. Not all doctors, however, are cut out to be clinical academics. In the past many SHOs felt compelled to undertake a higher degree to increase their chances of securing a national training number (NTN). While some were attracted to academia, for many this represented an unnecessary delay in their clinical training. It will still be possible for doctors to undertake higher degrees as part of their training, but it will no longer be required for clinical training.

To promote excellence and to recruit and retain those with the potential to be leaders in research and education, a clear career path has now been created for doctors wishing to become academics. These innovative training pathways were set out in the Walport report (*Medically and dentally qualified academic staff: Recommendations for training the researchers and educators of the future* (2005)).

> a clear **career path** has been created for **academics**

Figure 5 shows the new integrated training pathway, which is designed to take aspirant academics from foundation training through to CCT (or CESR) and to equip the academic with the necessary skills to take the lead in research.

The new integrated academic training pathway comprises two phases: academic clinical fellowship (ACF) and clinical lectureship (CL). The new

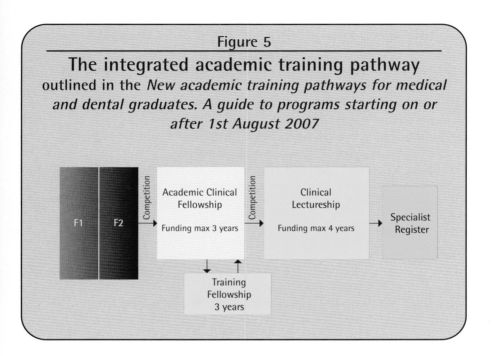

Figure 5

The integrated academic training pathway

outlined in the *New academic training pathways for medical and dental graduates. A guide to programs starting on or after 1st August 2007*

ACF is targeted at doctors in the early years of specialty training. It provides a clinical and academic training environment to help the academic clinical fellow prepare a competitive application for a training fellowship for a higher degree (e.g. Department of Health, Wellcome Trust, Medical Research Council) or if applicable a postdoctoral fellowship. Funding is available for a maximum of 3 years, or 4 years for GP academic clinical fellows. Further details are given on pages 23–39.

CL posts are designed for doctors with a PhD/MD (or equivalent), who already have some specialty training experience. They provide opportunities for research after a higher degree or educational training for doctors and dentists working towards completion of specialty training. Clinical lecturers are expected to apply for further research funding (e.g. personal fellowships or research grants), or support for continuing educational training. The CL phase ends with the award of a CCT or CESR. There are a number of different types of appointments for clinical academics including personal fellowships, clinician scientist awards, Higher Education Funding Council for England (HEFCE)-funded 'new blood' senior CLs, and university appointments.

Managing your medical career

These changes to postgraduate medical education and training are designed to enable you to develop the competences you require to be a safe and effective doctor. They are also designed to reduce the milling about that has characterized clinical training in the past.

To make best use of the opportunities provided, you should reflect on your aspirations and experiences. Discuss your interests with your clinical and educational supervisors and keep an eye open for new developments in clinical care. Research will no longer improve your chances of selection unless you are applying for the integrated academic training pathway. To progress and succeed, you must demonstrate that you have met the required standards of competence.

Good luck!

Further reading and resources

The Academy of Medical Royal Colleges can provide an up-to-date list of medical royal colleges and faculties
http://www.aomrc.org.uk/pages/links.htm

The Conference of Postgraduate Medical Education Deans of the UK provides details and web addresses of all postgraduate deaneries
http://www.copmed.org.uk/

Department of Health. *Curriculum for the foundation years in postgraduate education and training.* London: DH, 2005.
http://www.dh.gov.uk/assetRoot/04/10/76/96/04107696.pdf

Department of Health. *Good doctors, safer patients: Proposals to strengthen the system to assure and improve the performance of doctors and to protect the safety of patients. A report by the Chief Medical Officer.* 276071. London: DH, 2006.
http://www.dh.gov.uk/assetRoot/04/13/72/76/04137276.pdf

Department of Health (further information about postgraduate training)
http://www.dh.gov.uk/

General Medical Council (GMC) website has a section on education
http://www.gmc-uk.org/

General Medical Council. *Good Medical Practice.* London: GMC, 2006.
http://www.gmc-uk.org/guidance/good_medical_practice/index.asp

The Medical Training Application Service (MTAS) provides information about recruitment and selection processes foundation programmes, specialty training programmes and FTSTAs
http://www.mtas.nhs.uk/

Modernising Medical Careers website is at:
http://www.mmc.nhs.uk/

Modernising Medical Careers & UK Clinical Research Collaboration. *Medically and dentally qualified academic staff: Recommendations for training the researchers and educators of the future.* London: UKCRC, 2005.
http://www.ukcrc.org/PDF/Medically_and_Dentally-qualified_Academic_Staff_Report.pdf

Modernising Medical Careers & UK Clinical Research Collaboration. *New academic training pathways for medical and dental graduates, A guide to programs starting on or after 1st August 2007.* London: DH, 2006.
http://www.mmc.nhs.uk/download_files/A-pocket-guide.pdf

Modernising Medical Careers. *Operational framework for foundation training.* London: DH, 2005.
http://www.mmc.nhs.uk/download_files/Operational-Framework.pdf

Mumford C. *The Medical Job Interview: Secrets for Success,* 2nd edn. Oxford: Blackwell, 2005.

National Confidential Enquiry into Perioperative Deaths (now National Confidential Enquiry into Patient Outcome and Death). *Changing the way we operate: The 2001 Report of the National Confidential Enquiry into Perioperative Deaths.* London: NCEPOD, 2001.
http://www.ncepod.org.uk/2001.htm

The National Co-ordinating Centre for Research Capacity Development provides information about the new integrated academic training pathway
http://www.nccrcd.nhs.uk/

Postgraduate Medical Education and Training Board (PMETB) explains the routes to certification
http://www.pmetb.org.uk/

research

John D Kelly
Department of Oncology, University of Cambridge

*'Where observation is concerned, chance
favours only the prepared mind'*
Louis Pasteur (1822–1895)

At trainee level

Research in the field of clinical medicine, biological and health sciences affords an opportunity for intellectual stimulation and personal development. For us doctors, the drive for evidence through research is part of our psyche and intellect and cannot be easily separated from the conduct of our day-to-day professional life. Despite this, research is regarded by many as a means to career progression, so perhaps it is best viewed as a process in which personal development and career development go hand in hand. Fortunately there are now a number of routes by which trainees can engage in research activity and thus develop both themselves and their careers.

The changes brought about through Modernising Medical Careers (MMC; see pages 3–22) will undoubtedly affect the way trainees and, for that matter, appointment panels perceive the requirement to conduct full-time research within the context of what will soon be a structured career pathway. It is likely that the selection criteria for specialist training will no longer follow the old dogma that a postgraduate degree is necessary. Instead, academic training posts will be available for those who wish to undertake research because they genuinely want to conduct experimental or clinical studies to find out more about, or make a breakthrough in, a particular subject. Two new academic training appointments have been designed for trainees with an interest in an academic career, namely an academic clinical fellowship (ACF) and a clinical lectureship (CL), both with an 'academic' national training number (NTNA). The ACF can be held for a period of 3 years, during which the trainee will spend a portion of the working week developing a research project with the aim of obtaining pilot data and applying for funding to begin a period of full-time research likely to culminate in a PhD. Having completed the postgraduate degree, the clinical fellow will be eligible for an academic clinical lecturer position permitting a 50:50 timetable split between clinical and research duties.

entry to **fellowships** will be **highly competitive**

In practice the number of trainees likely to follow this route will be limited, and those who wish to pursue an academic career will self-select. Entry will be highly competitive, as the number of Fellowships will be restricted, and the trainee who attains a Fellowship has in one sense already mapped out a career structure beyond completion of their training through to Lecturer and to an academic Chair.

However, many trainees wish to become involved in research at a level which does not require career commitment but enables participation in a project, perhaps as part of a scientific or clinical research team, leading to a publication or a degree such as MSc. By involvement at this level, you will gain experience in searching the literature, assessing conflicting results and opinions, and interpreting what you read. You will also learn scientific methodology and the use of particular techniques – having first-hand experience inevitably makes it easier to assess the results of others. And, of course, you will have the opportunity to have papers published in peer-reviewed journals and to present your work at national and international meetings. Furthermore, in this time you can develop your skills in working with a team, thinking strategically and managing your time effectively. It is very likely that future training schemes will facilitate structured career breaks for such research activity with provision for trainees holding a national training number (NTN) to undertake a period of full-time research culminating in an MD or perhaps PhD. In reality there will always be a competitive selection pressure for posts at consultant level within the UK, and many trainees will develop their CVs with the aim of being appointed as, for example, an NHS Consultant in academic institution or a large teaching hospital. The system now being rolled out aims on the one hand to foster top-level academic appointments and on the other to encourage and facilitate research at many levels, but removes the postdoctoral degree as an unnecessary hurdle to specialist training. The key is to plan ahead and think about your long-term aspirations; although these may change, it is easier to step down than to step up.

plan ahead and think about your **long-term aspirations**

Defining your research

The first step is to decide which research route you want to pursue; whether you want to apply for a clinical fellowship or consider an MSc or MD if you already hold an NTN; and whether you want to conduct clinical research as part of your training with a view to a high-quality publication. These decisions will be in some way based on your track record as an undergraduate, your enthusiasm for a specialist subject and the environment within which you are working. Be clear about the reasons for selecting an option and how it fits with your future plans.

Committing to a project

It is most important that you avoid a research trap that exists at all levels from clinical case reporting to basic scientific projects. Without careful planning and a willingness to challenge, it is possible to become involved in a project that requires 90% of your effort to deliver a 10% output. The natural history of such projects is that they fail to complete; they are time-consuming and frequently do nothing other than restate what is already known and are therefore not worthy of a significant publication. The typical scenario is the discussion over coffee, a case series begging to be written up, perhaps a biological question which needs addressing. These are the informal discussions that are part of our professional profile; they are stimulating and often exciting, but read around the subject carefully before you commit. Find out whether the research has been done previously – summarize the

read around the subject carefully **before you commit**

> ### Table 2
> ## Profile of a good supervisor
>
> **A good supervisor:**
> - Is interested in what you are doing
> - Has the time and inclination to help you to do it
> - Has facilities at his or her disposal and is able to draw on the expertise of others to help in areas where he or she cannot help you or at times when he or she is unavailable
> - Will say what he or she thinks without equivocation and give useful advice and direction
> - Will check your written work carefully, correct it and provide further guidance when necessary
> - Will motivate you to complete the project

literature and present findings to a potential supervisor, or better still at a departmental meeting; this will also help you focus on the work you intend to do. Many aspects of good-quality research develop this way, and the enthusiasm of a trainee to take on the challenge is rarely dampened.

It is particularly important to find a supervisor who will oversee your project from start to finish and ensure that you benefit from your research experience (Table 2). If you are not in the right place with the right people and the right facilities, then you may have to go elsewhere or modify your plans to fit the location. An informal face-to-face meeting with a potential supervisor will pay a lot more dividends than a letter or circulated CV (the latter is pretty much a waste of time).

Getting started

If you decide to pursue a period of full-time research and you have identified a supervisor with a track record and a group which has a focus and drive that fits your requirements, then start to develop a written proposal or protocol for your intended research. This should include:
- a clear description of the aims and objectives and a statement of the hypothesis you want to test (one way to test your aims is to

formulate a null hypothesis: will your aims enable you to reject the null hypothesis?)
- a critical review and a justification of your study based on your literature review
- a reasonably detailed outline of the proposed study:
  - your research goal and how you are going to achieve it
  - the timeline
  - pilot data that support the work and show that your goals are achievable
- the statistical methodology that you are going to use to interpret your results.

If the work involves human subjects or human tissues or if it affects patients, you will need to submit your proposal to an ethics committee or to the trust's research committee for approval. Few trainees would be expected to undertake this task single-handed. The process is an administrative minefield; if your supervisor has little experience of ethics submissions, be careful about proceeding.

When you have finished an outline research draft, scrutinize it and improve it. Give it to a colleague whose opinion you respect to read.

You should then obtain an expert opinion and appropriate statistical guidance from your supervisor. Most hospitals have a statistics expert available who will be able to help you to ensure that your study has the best possible chance of producing meaningful results. Nowadays, there are many good statistical software packages available. When you have a supervisor-approved protocol, you can submit it to the appropriate bodies. Bear in mind that they may want revisions made and may even turn down a revised proposal. Nonetheless, if you have a good supervisor, you should be able to get it right eventually.

There is often a phase between submission of a grant or ethical committee application and receiving a reply when it appears that there is nothing much to do. Actually there is quite a lot to do. In particular, this time may be used for reading to

Time is a non-renewable resource – don't waste it

ensure that, when your experimental study begins, the majority of background reading has been done. If it is a clinical study then you can begin to recruit patients, which is always more difficult and time-consuming than you think it will be at the outset, irrespective of your subject. Patients can be identified and approached informally before an ethics committee has given formal approval. If it is laboratory research, then you can start to familiarize yourself with techniques and instrumentation, either directly or by watching others work. Time is the most valuable commodity and a non-renewable resource – don't waste it!

Practical points

When you perform your research, whether a clinical study or laboratory investigation, make sure everybody concerned knows what you are doing and why you are doing it. You may need help and advice, and you will certainly not want to be forgotten! Coming into a laboratory environment can be somewhat unnerving. You immediately sense that your skill mix is not applicable and you can feel that you are back at the beginning. This is not the case! Your medical training has developed your skills as a team player and communicator; you can rapidly assimilate information and solve problems. These, together with the intellectual challenge, will enable you to integrate into the team. But beware: focus on the job in hand, learn the do's and don'ts of laboratory life. Once you start to work independently don't flit from idea to idea like a butterfly!

don't flit from **idea** to **idea**

As you work, it is important to document all you do – make duplicate copies whenever you can and back up computer files onto removable media regularly. If possible, obtain a state-of-the-art laptop computer and install software for statistics and compiling references. Equally important, start to write up your project at the earliest possible opportunity, as it always takes longer than you think. When you are not actively researching, write. All too often, research is completed before writing up begins: the funding runs out and the researcher takes a clinical

start to **write up** at the **earliest** possible **opportunity** job and no longer has the time to write up. It is tragic to contemplate how much good-quality research never sees the light of day for this reason, and the number of careers that are marred by the failure to deliver the results of their research.

Funding at more senior level

Senior research is a serious business that requires serious money. The expense of starting a new study and the uncertainties of funding are such that research is always best carried out in a department with a track record in that particular area, in which equipment, expertise and experience already exist.

Research departments exist on the grant income that they raise both directly and indirectly. Directly, a grant will pay the salaries of most of the people who work in the department, apart from the fortunate, but increasingly rare, senior scientists with tenured appointments funded by the department until they retire. Indirectly, the level and source of funding constitute the means by which university department review committees assess research departments, such as the Research Assessment Exercise (RAE) conducted by the Higher Education Funding Council for England (HEFCE). A £50 000 grant from the Medical Research Council (MRC) or the Wellcome Trust (awarded after a competitive peer-review process) may be considered by the RAE to be more prestigious than £100 000 from an anonymous private donor.

The first step is to decide whether the research to be undertaken is of sufficient scientific merit to attract the interest of one of the major grant-giving bodies. If so, the next step is to approach the most appropriate body or bodies and obtain a copy of their instructions to applicants; these are available on the websites of the major funding bodies. Many of the larger funding bodies also issue annual reports that list the organization's research priorities – you should be able to find out whether your planned research is in one of the areas generally funded. Some also welcome informal applications to discuss a proposal before formal submission. Generally speaking, pilot data in support of your application are essential, and only a group with a research track and funding stream can help you generate data.

Clinical research

The main source of funding for clinically orientated research is the NHS Research and Development Initiative, the principal aim of which is to develop the database necessary for sound decisions on health policy. Health Technology Assessment is the largest of the programmes within this initiative, and its research priorities are identified and published by the Standing Group on Health Technology.

Laboratory-based research

The leading body for funding laboratory research (although also involved in health services research) is the MRC. It provides a wide range of grants, not only for individual studies, but also for training fellowships and travel grants for work in overseas departments. As well as clinical lectureships, the MRC and Cancer Research UK (CRUK) will fund Clinician Scientists, enabling you to continue your career as a consultant in academic medicine or surgery. This level of award is available to trainees who have been awarded a PhD and in some circumstances an MD. For non-cancer-related research, the Wellcome Trust is the major funding body. It tends to be less molecular-biology orientated and encourages informal approaches in the first instance to verify whether formal applications are appropriate. Otherwise it functions in much the same way as the MRC.

A number of other large charities concentrate on specific diseases, for example the British Heart Foundation, the Arthritis and Rheumatism Council and the National Kidney Research Fund. Each of these, like the MRC, offers several different types of grant. A list of charities that fund medical research in relation to particular diseases outside these areas can be found in the *Association of Medical Research Charities Handbook* (see Useful addresses, page 231).

European funding

The European Commission is becoming increasingly important in funding research. Its contributions include those of the European Community Research and Development Programme, which is comparable to the NHS Research and Development Initiative, and those of the Economic and Social Research Council, which is comparable to the MRC, although its primary fields of interest are psychology- and sociology-based studies.

Alternative funding bodies

There are other, albeit less prestigious, sources of funding for research. The most widely used are the local charities affiliated to hospital trusts. Larger charities, such as the British Heart Foundation and the MS Society, also sponsor significant amounts of research. Their application procedures are generally less formal, although still rigorous. Many smaller charities and trusts also offer grants for research focussed on their own area of interest.

Professional societies such as the Royal Colleges have funds available for research grants, often in the form of fellowships, which are only marginally less prestigious than those from the major grant-giving bodies.

Most major drug companies and medical equipment manufacturers sponsor medical research. Indeed, in the UK, pharmaceutical-company-sponsored research overall is currently the largest contributor to medical research. Much of this 'soft money' is dedicated to the development and marketing of new drugs, but some may be awarded as a fellowship for more altruistic purposes, in which case similar application procedures will apply. Getting these grants is

always **maintain** the highest
ethical standards

often quicker and easier than going through the traditional funding bodies. When submitting a proposal for such a grant, remember the 'What's in it for them?' principle. Pharmaceutical companies are businesses and are unlikely to sponsor projects that do not reflect the general direction in which they are heading. Be sure that the work you perform for them, and others, always maintains probity and the highest ethical standards.

Non-medical funding bodies

There are research councils, other than the MRC, relevant to those in medical research, particularly in biomaterials or biotechnology. Organizations such as the Engineering and Physical Sciences Research

Council (EPSRC) and the Biotechnology and Biological Sciences Research Council (BBSRC) function in much the same way as the MRC and produce their own handbooks outlining the grants and awards available.

The Department of Trade and Industry (http://www.dti.gov.uk/) funds six LINK programmes in healthcare to promote collaboration between university departments and industry. These are particularly appropriate for those engaged in research likely to produce new technology that has the potential to be developed commercially by the industrial partner.

Types of grant

The most common type of grant from the bodies described above is the project grant. A project grant is designed to support a specific study by covering the salary of a full-time research assistant for 2–3 years, together with the costs of the research study itself in terms of equipment and consumables. Such grants run to tens of thousands of pounds.

Rather more prestigious is a programme grant that covers the cost of a large-scale study by supporting a research team and its associated costs rather than just an individual. These often run to hundreds of thousands of pounds. Very few of these grants are awarded each year and it is the pinnacle of a researcher's ambition to receive one – an award deemed only slightly lower than winning a Nobel Prize! Only a team of experienced researchers could expect to receive a programme grant. If you are a trainee seeking an appropriate environment in which to conduct research, groups and institutions holding programme grants are likely to offer the range of skills, technologies and support that will enable your project to succeed.

Grant applications

All grants are awarded after intense competitive scrutiny. Grant application writing is an arduous process (indeed, many universities have departments dedicated to helping researchers produce grant applications) and most applications submitted are likely to be rejected. The principles are the same as those for preparing an outline proposal at a junior level, but should be applied much more rigorously.

- The application must outline the purpose of the study.
- The need for new research in this area should be supported by a brief literature review.

- The aims must be clearly outlined, indicating the potential benefits of the study.
- The intended methodology, including data to be collected and statistical techniques for analysis, must be fully described.
- Study requirements must be stated and justified in detail. These will include salaries for research staff, essential equipment and running costs, including consumables, and other expenses such as travel and subsistence to present research results.

Funding bodies usually, but not always, have a specific application form on which to present this information, although some – like the Wellcome Trust – prefer an informal written approach in the first instance; they will forward an application form if the proposal is of interest. Be aware that your grant application has to be scrutinized by the research services division of your university. This process usually requires the application to be submitted at least one, possibly two, weeks ahead of the official deadline. Funding bodies will reject delayed applications, so plan ahead and discuss timelines with your supervisor and administrators.

All funding bodies have a similar assessment process to deal with applications. They have a grants committee to review applications that includes their own experts and external referees with expertise in the particular subject area. At least two, and often more, external referees will review and individually rate each application. A group of applications will then be considered together by the committee. Competition is such that all applications are likely to be of an extremely high standard, so only those with an alpha plus or similar rating from the internal and external referees are likely to be accepted, and even these cannot assume success.

Each applicant, therefore, needs to convince the reviewers that his or her application poses an important research question, will use appropriate and feasible research methodology, and if possible that the study will be conducted by researchers with experience in that particular area. Commonly, applications are unsuccessful because the research question is unimportant and/or poorly presented, or the research methodology or analytical techniques are inappropriate or imprecise. Occasionally, there may be insufficient experience or expertise in the research team to bring the research to a satisfactory conclusion.

The key to success is a well-prepared, clear and concise application. If a previous application has been submitted or if preliminary advice has been sought from the funding body, take notice of any criticisms and comments, and ensure that the application is put together carefully, allowing plenty of time to write, rewrite and rewrite again if necessary.

> allow plenty of **time** to **write, rewrite** and **rewrite** again

Follow the application instructions supplied by the funding body closely and seek advice from those with experience in writing grant applications. Read through the application in detail and remove any excess or inappropriate text. Most important of all, don't be surprised or disappointed if your first application is turned down. Writing a successful grant application is an academic goal in its own right.

Writing up

The principles involved in writing a thesis or preparing a paper for publication in a journal are essentially the same. In the first instance, you should decide for whom you are writing and find out what rules and regulations apply. These are available from universities, in the case of theses, or from the journal to which you intend to submit your paper. The general format is an initial summary followed by an introduction, materials and methods, results and discussion sections. For a thesis, the introduction is usually a detailed historical literature review of the general subject together with an outline of the question under consideration and another detailed relevant literature review specific to the study question. Whatever the nature of your publication, it will be reviewed by at least two experts in the field who will be familiar with, and may well have contributed to, the relevant literature. They will be aware of the difficulties that exist in your particular area of research and will expect to see adequate coverage of the potential sources of error in your study in the discussion section. Equally important to a critical analysis of potential sources of error is the future relevance of any research findings. Which questions remain unanswered, and where should future research be directed to develop further the implications of your study?

Aim to have as much as possible written up before completing your research, though data analysis will need to wait until all the results are available. Write as you go along, and as soon as you have finished a first draft give it to somebody else to read. Expect them to tear it to shreds – this is all part of the learning process. Use this criticism constructively; it is preferable for your supervisor to point out defects in your work in private than for an examiner or an audience to do so during a viva or at a major national or international meeting. Such criticism should not be taken as a personal insult, but instead viewed as helpful feedback.

Remember that when you have completed a piece of research you will automatically be one of the world's leading authorities on that very narrow topic. Indeed, unless you have simply repeated somebody else's specific investigation, you will be the leading authority on the subject, at least for a brief time. Therefore, others will criticize you (in the strictest sense of the word), not so much about what you have done

> the **most important** part of published **research** is the **critical self-analysis**

but on how you have done it. The most important part of published research, to the critical reader, is the critical self-analysis in the discussion section. Analyse all potential sources of error in the conclusions you have derived from your results, particularly with reference to methodology. When examining your thesis, the examiner will probably concentrate on how you have critically reviewed the literature in the first chapter and your analysis of results in the discussion section later on. Your results – although probably dearest to your heart – will often be less important to the examiner than your interpretation of them.

Statistical work, particularly involving clinical evaluation of patients, should be presented very carefully and reviewed following guidelines such as those laid down in the BMJ. Statistical advice should have been sought before the project began to ensure that no problems would come to light at this late stage.

In short, research involves a great deal of work, but most people appreciate it or learn something from it, and hopefully both.

Finally, writing up is the most demanding part of completing a research project, and many people present their work at meetings but never complete the thesis or get the papers published. Failing to

> **Failing** to **write up** marks you out as a **non-completer**

'make the conversion' marks you out as a non-completer and acts as a permanent millstone around your neck.

Supervising a research project

If you are supervising a research project that is being conducted by others, you should aim to fulfil the criteria that you expected of your supervisor when you were the junior partner. It is a good idea to hold weekly meetings at which every researcher in the team presents their results and progress to date, and which provide an opportunity for constructive critical appraisal by colleagues. In addition, meet with each researcher to discuss their work to date and monitor progress against the project timetable that has been set within the constraints of time and funding. In particular, ensure that the research is written up and that each draft is handed to you to read through; give constructive criticism

hold **weekly meetings** at which every researcher **presents** results and **progress**

and comments, and set a deadline for submission of each revised draft until you are satisfied with the final copy.

Finally, identify any interesting ideas for future research so that, if possible, these can be developed by a subsequent researcher. You are likely to be acknowledged in his or her publications and you may be able to maintain valuable long-term contact with the institution.

Projects sponsored by pharmaceutical companies

The pharmaceutical industry is the main source of research funding in the UK overall. Unlike the major grant-giving bodies and private donors, who normally respond to a research proposal, pharmaceutical companies direct the research they sponsor; the researcher's responsibility is to manage the project. In most instances, the pharmaceutical company will determine the objectives of the study, although there is sometimes opportunity for discussion of the details. Indeed, you are likely to have been approached because of your particular expertise in the field.

It is important not to underestimate the potential financial value of your research in pharmaceutical-company-sponsored projects, nor to overestimate its intellectual value. In any project, most of the benefit comes from planning the patient selection methodology and, in particular, the statistical assessment and analysis of results. In research sponsored by pharmaceutical companies, the company usually performs the analysis when data from individual patient studies are sent back to it. Carefully consider the time that you will need to invest before embarking on such a project. Before committing yourself, ask around to find out the going rate so that you are in a position to negotiate and ensure that you are not undervalued. Be aware that there is intense financial pressure to generate accurate data and results within a defined time.

If you do take part in clinical trials, or indeed any other research enlisting patients or volunteers, you are responsible for ensuring that each patient understands clearly the implications and has given written, informed consent for their involvement in the trial, and that the research is not contrary to their interests. You should always seek further advice in cases where individuals are not capable of making informed decisions for themselves and, in particular, if you are undertaking research that involves children. Always be sure to check that a properly constituted research ethics committee has approved every aspect of the research protocol.

Avoiding the pitfalls

Remember to ask yourself at every step 'is this piece of research ethical?' If in any doubt, ask the advice of your supervisor or someone more senior, and always have your research approved by the appropriate ethical committee. If your research involves the storage and use of human tissue, including DNA, make yourself acquainted with the Human Tissue Act of 2004; this makes removal and storage of organs without consent an offence. For more information, see the document *Research: The role and responsibilities of doctors*, available on the GMC website (http://www.gmc-uk.org).

If the research involves a clinical trial, make sure that the foreseeable risks and inconveniences have been weighed against the anticipated benefit for the individual trial subject and other present and future patients. A trial should only be initiated and continued if the anticipated benefits justify the risks. The rights, safety and wellbeing of the trial subjects are the most important considerations and should prevail over the interests of science and society (Table 3). After a clinical trial went badly wrong in Northwick Park in 2006, leaving six individuals in intensive care, the issue of truly informed consent of research subjects has been highlighted. Any individual you invite to take part in research must be given the information that they ought to know, presented in terms and a form that they can understand. You must bear in mind that it may be difficult for participants to genuinely identify and assess the risks involved. Giving the information will require an initial discussion supported by a patient information sheet or sound recording in a form and language that they can understand. You must give participants an opportunity to ask questions and express any concerns they may have.

Table 3

When designing or carrying out research

- Put the participants' interests first
- Act with honesty and integrity
- Follow the appropriate national research governance guidelines and the GMC guidance

---

In conclusion, research can and should be both fulfilling and tremendous fun, but does require the researcher to be an honest, hard-working self-starter and a diligent completer of tasks. However, beware the temptation to make your results fit the hypothesis. This must be resisted sternly, as integrity and probity in research is just as essential as in clinical medicine.

Further reading and resources

Baxter L, Hughes C, Tight M. *How to Research*. Buckingham: Open University Press, 1996.

Benatar D, Benatar SR. Informed consent and research. *BMJ* 1998;316:1008.

Department of Health. *Research Governance Framework for Health and Social Care.* London: DH, 2005.
http://www.dh.gov.uk

General Medical Council. *Research: the role and responsibilities of doctors.* London: GMC, 2002.
http://www.gmc-uk.org/guidance/current/library/research.asp

Medical Research Council. *Ethics and Research Governance.* London: MRC, 2006.
http://www.mrc.ac.uk/PolicyGuidance/EthicsAndGovernance/index.htm

Murrell G, Huang C, Ellis H. *Research in Medicine: Planning a Project – Writing a Thesis.* 2nd edn. Cambridge: Cambridge University Press, 1999.

Power L. Trial subjects must be fully involved in design and approval of trials. *BMJ* 1998;316:1003–4.

making your mark
in the NHS

'Seek opportunity, not security. A boat in a harbour
is safe, but in time its bottom will rot out'
Life's Little Instruction Book, H Jackson Brown Jr (1991)

So your post is secured. You have reached the first real postqualification high point – you are a consultant. But beware! This is the point at which many doctors find themselves becoming somewhat disillusioned. With no obvious goals to achieve, many experience a form of anxiety and/or depression. So, how can you maintain and build on your initial success?

Striving for continued success

Others (generally statutory bodies) have set the goals that you have achieved to date, but now you should begin to set your own goals. Indeed, setting and attaining personal goals is fundamental to your success as a consultant in the NHS – just as it is in any walk of life.

You must also appreciate the importance of change in clinical practice as well as in everyday life. Now that you no longer have examinations and superiors to make sure you develop, you yourself will have to seek out reasons to modify your practice and take responsibility for making the necessary improvements. Most importantly, do not allow yourself to become complacent and out of touch; you will get left behind.

The last general point concerns your life outside medicine. Non-medical partners or spouses tend to assume that when you get to the top of the ladder – that is, you become a consultant – you will not have to work so hard: your on-call duties will diminish, you will not have to stay late in the hospital every evening and so on. But you do not have to be a consultant for very long to know that this is untrue. In some instances you will spend less time on call, but even so, this extra time will be more than compensated for by the enormous amount of extra paperwork, management and general clinical responsibility that a consultant takes on as the leader, or one of the leaders, of a clinical team. It is important then to remember your family and, in particular, that nobody on their deathbed ever says, 'I wish I had spent more time at work'. Look after yourself and your family – you should take care of your own health and your family's well-being, and not allow yourself to become estranged from your friends and loved ones. Try to find a focus for your free time, ideally something that you can share with your family. There are few things as boring as a consultant who comes home and immediately burrows into some paperwork or starts up the laptop, and talks about nothing but work. For goodness' sake, avoid this at all costs! As Brian Dyson, CEO of the Pepsi Cola Corporation, wrote: 'Imagine life as a game in which you are juggling five balls in the air. You name them work, family, friends, health and spirit. You will soon learn that work is a rubber ball; if you drop it, it will bounce back. But the other four are made of glass; if you drop them they will be irrevocably damaged or even shattered. You must understand this to achieve the right balance in your life.' Achieving personal happiness and maintaining quality family relationships and friendships are just as important as building a successful career, and part of becoming an overall success.

Don't forget also the sensible financial planning is important. Doctors tend to assume that money will accrue automatically, but good, independent financial advice is invaluable. It is hard to be a successful doctor if you and your family are undermined by constant financial pressures.

This is clearly not the place to tell readers how to achieve personal and family happiness; nor are the authors best placed to define this. However, it is worth mentioning that divorce is more common in medicine than in many other walks of life. Most doctors know of colleagues who have got into 'difficulties' trying to balance the competing demands of a medical career and a family. Choosing a supportive and encouraging partner is the first step. Even so, moments of stress will arise, especially as children come along. As with all aspects of life, it is easier to find a way through if you

> nobody ever says, 'I wish I had spent more time at work'

anticipate and talk about the problems, rather than sweeping them under the carpet or dealing with them when it is already too late. Seeking advice from somebody outside the immediate situation can also be invaluable. Once you appreciate that you are stressed, that stress can be managed more easily.

Women have the added difficulty of fitting childbearing around their training. In the past, many women who wished to have a family used to wait until they had become consultants before having children. Nowadays, it is more usual to elect to have 'flexible training', allowing training and motherhood to run concurrently. Deaneries have a designated flexible training coordinator to provide advice on such matters. Training committees should be sympathetic to the aspirations of all trainees – men as well as women – who want to undergo flexible training. Regardless of the stage at which children appear, they need to be incorporated into the 'grand plan' and that is best considered in advance. Job sharing, for example, is a option that many have found helpful.

Finding your focus

The single largest problem when finding your focus, setting goals and yet maintaining a healthy and rewarding life outside medicine is time. Generally, the most successful people are those who manage their time, and themselves, most effectively (see pages 46–48). Furthermore, because medicine involves dealing with people, either as patients or colleagues, successful individuals relate well to other people, often enlisting the help of others to enable them to use their time efficiently. Successful consultants know what they are going to do and how they

> **successful people manage** their **time**, and themselves, **effectively**

are going to do it; they set themselves objectives towards a final goal (and then maybe a further goal when that one has been achieved). Making the best of time and people usually means building a good team that functions happily, efficiently and effectively. When the team is in place, delegate work appropriately and reward those who do it with praise and recognition for their efforts.

Taking control

As a new consultant, the first thing you must do is determine how you will fulfil your contractual obligation of fixed and flexible sessions and on-call commitments. These vary from post to post, and will be clearly stated in the consultant job plan. Then you must establish how you are going to carry out your clinical practice, fulfil teaching commitments and conduct any planned research. Other aspects to consider include:

- establishing and running your own office
- developing a good working relationship with your secretary
- ensuring that you have sufficient junior staff and equipment.

Of these, the first two are particularly important. Equipment and trainees are usually provided or allocated by other agencies, but establishing an efficient office with a good secretary is very much a personal concern. It is important to develop a routine so that people know what you do and when, and when you can or cannot be interrupted or contacted. Allow yourself protected time during the week to think, plan, reflect, and deal with paperwork and other routine management issues. Also, set aside time for informal discussion and let your colleagues know when you will be available.

At this stage, it is helpful to obtain advice, whether you feel you need it or not, from others who have been through the same experience already. What do they do and how do they do it? It is certainly not a weakness to ask for opinions and advice, and learning from the experience of others can save a great deal of time and prevent mistakes. Reading this book, of course, is a step in the right direction!

> it is **not** a **weakness** to **ask** for **advice**

Increasing your clinical expertise

On a clinical level, it is important to keep up to date with your specialty, not only by reading, but also by discussing clinical problems you encounter with the people you regard as your peers or those with greater expertise than yourself. The smaller your focus of interest becomes, the more difficult this may be. It has been said that experience allows you to recognize a mistake the next time you make it (and also that good judgement results from experience, which results from bad judgement), but you can also learn from the mistakes of others.

Make sure that those you would like to regard as your peers are aware of your particular interest, and try to establish yourself as an authority in that area. Attend seminars and conferences in your chosen field – show your face and stand up to speak at appropriate opportunities to underline your interest. Publish as much as you can in that area, making sure that your publications are of the highest quality, clearly presented and relevant to others. Remember, though, when you write something you adopt a particular position, and later the view you took may come back to haunt you, as often happens in politics!

> We are **drowning** in **information,** but **thirsting** for **knowledge**

Keeping up to date

Some doctors become dissatisfied with medicine for a number of reasons: too much work and not enough time to do it; a declining income in real terms (as they see it); increasing medicolegal liability; anger, frustration, depression and a feeling of loss of control of their job and future. The issue most commonly cited, however, is information overload. There is simply too much being published and too much to know. It has been aptly said, 'We are drowning in information, but thirsting for knowledge.' Dealing with the volume of information and retrieving what you need to know is an essential skill that you will need to acquire.

The first step is to think about how this applies to you. Time spent planning strategically and reflecting is always valuable; decide what you need to know, where it can be found and how you are going to learn it or have it available. It is impossible to keep up to date with everything, so deciding what you actually need to know is vital.

Most people have piles of journals and unread material littering their office and home. It usually remains unread because most of it does not need to be read. So establish what needs to be read, photocopy, scan (an excellent option if you have a flat-bed scanner) or otherwise file it, and discard the journal. Having filed it, make sure that you can retrieve it readily when necessary. Learning to use modern information technology is particularly valuable in this regard. Online journal databases, such as PubMed and Medline, provide an invaluable means of keeping up to date on subjects that you need to know about while avoiding irrelevant subjects. You can also have the satisfaction of seeing your own publication list grow online!

Throughout your medical training and subsequent career, invest in yourself by focusing on your own continuing professional development, attitudes and interpersonal skills, and appraise them constantly. These are just as important as the more traditional scientific skills and knowledge. Be a self-starter. Be prepared to state in an appraisal which research or audit projects you have initiated and seen through to completion and publication; choose examples which illustrate imagination, innovation and flair. Mention things that have actually changed for the better as a result of your own input and drive.

Managing your time

It has been estimated that 80% of a person's productivity is a result of 20% of their time. If true, this means that most of our time is wasted. Some people are perfectionists and will achieve less because of their quest for perfection in everything they do; on balance, efficiency is better than perfection for most purposes, and becomes all the more important as your workload increases. Remember, though, that people tend to forget the thousand things you did well, but remember vividly and often talk about your solitary mistake. Therefore be diligent, indeed obsessive, about the things that count, especially patient safety!

efficiency is better than perfection

Set priorities, paying particular attention to tasks that only you can perform, and adhere to them. One of the most important management skills to acquire is successful delegation. If someone else could do a task as well as or better than you, then delegate it, and don't forget to thank the person who does it for you and, most importantly, give him or her the credit for the achievement.

To use your time efficiently, never start something that you are not going to finish and always complete one task before moving on to the next. Don't postpone an unpleasant or boring task – it will never improve with time – but do avoid starting anything when you are bored, miserable, tired or unable to focus and put in the effort required. Most people work most efficiently in the morning, so allocate some quality time first thing when interruptions are unlikely, and get the job done.

You should also think about the bigger picture and spend time developing your own personal strategy. Decide what your goals are and set yourself a realistic time frame within which to achieve them. Divide major tasks into smaller, more achievable parts and tick them off your list one by one. Review and update the list regularly and ask yourself why certain things seem harder to deal with than others (for example launching a website – do you need expert assistance?). Consider the potential pitfalls and identify what your key focus areas should be. Regularly take the time to think about your strategy and constantly modify it as individual goals are achieved.

Paperwork

Avoid wasting time on pointless paperwork. Always deal with paperwork first thing in the day, and follow a general rule to deal with it once and once only. The two exceptions to this rule are matters that need to be addressed at a later date when more information becomes available, and documents that require serious reading in peace and quiet before you reply.

When you pick up an item, your response to it should be one of the following:
- dictate a reply
- pass it to a more appropriate person to deal with
- delegate it to your secretary
- delegate it to someone within your team
- throw it in the rubbish bin.

Telephone calls

Making telephone calls is another potential waste of time. Our experience suggests you may have only a one in four chance of reaching the person you want to speak to. If possible, get someone else to make calls on your behalf and have them put calls through to you when the person you wish to speak to is on the line. Better still, use faxes, text messages or e-mail and ensure that incoming fax and e-mail messages are brought to your attention immediately. Mobile devices such as the BlackBerry™ allow you to communicate electronically when you are on the move and abroad, and can dramatically improve your overall efficiency. E-mails are a great bugbear these days, but dealing with them swiftly, efficiently, and politely is the hallmark of a successful person. Do not allow them to build up; allocate time to sort them effectively, and beware the flippant or jocular remark. E-mail is a very public communication medium, and an indiscretion may well come back to haunt you!

Committees

It is always flattering to be asked to join a committee, but is your presence really needed? If not, politely decline the invitation. One of the first principles of efficiency is learning to say no – politely, indirectly perhaps, but firmly. If your timetable is busy, don't join another committee or add another regular commitment until you can drop something that you are already involved with. Don't let others set your agenda for you; be your own man or woman.

Being assertive and staying in control

Learning to say 'no' is important, but being assertive is certainly not the same as being aggressive. To be assertive, you must be clear in your own mind what you want and be ready and able to express your opinion clearly and politely. You should always try to offer advice, information and solutions to problems rather than just complaining about them. If you do not understand something, be prepared to ask for clarification and advice or information from others when you need it.

Inevitably, assertion and aggression interrelate when you have to confront someone behaving wrongly or inappropriately, but in almost every instance you can, and should, manage such situations without aggression. Above all, always try to stay in control not only of yourself but also of the situation you find yourself in.

Working as part of a team

Doctors can have some rather unfortunate characteristics. Younger ones tend to be aloof and arrogant, older ones cranky, and both tend to be rather paternalistic. Some can be verbally abusive and sarcastic in public, and some even argue openly, which can be embarrassing and cruel to those on the receiving end. None of the above is an attractive trait. As a senior member of staff, you should set the standard of professional and social behaviour that everyone else follows.

Involve everyone in your decisions, be considerate to your co-workers and give credit when it is due. Remember that today's trainees are tomorrow's colleagues. Furthermore, to delegate effectively you will need to have a good relationship with your team members, not one based on humiliation and abuse. Remember that those you stab in the back on your way up the ladder may get their revenge when you are on the way down!

If you work in a team, as most of us do nowadays, always take into account the others in the group and the way in which they interact (Table 4). The people you work with deserve your full confidence, and they should know that they have it. If someone interacts badly within the group or with a patient, take that person aside and discuss the matter

Table 4
Working in teams

- Respect the skills and contributions of your colleagues
- Communicate effectively with colleagues inside and outside the team
- Make sure that your patients and colleagues understand your role and responsibilities in the team and know who is responsible for each aspect of patient care
- Participate in regular reviews and audit of the standards and performance of the team, taking steps to remedy any deficiencies
- Support colleagues who have problems with performance, conduct or health

Adapted from General Medical Council. *Good Medical Practice* London: GMC, 2006.
http://www.gmc-uk.org/guidance/good_medical_practice/index.asp

with him or her (with the aim of ensuring that the situation does not happen again). In this way, you can develop your team and your leadership of that team. Remember that your team is an extension of yourself and if an incident reflects badly on them, it also reflects badly on you.

give **credit** when it is **due**

Regardless of who you are dealing with, it is always best to say what you think, tactfully, having thought the matter through thoroughly so that you are certain of your opinion. Some people are reluctant and embarrassed to say what they think, while others are inclined to say what the listener would like to hear, irrespective of what they really think. Ultimately, neither of these approaches is satisfactory. It is easiest and best to state a problem clearly and give your view about its solution, whether you are advising a junior about his or her training or a consultant colleague about a clinical issue. This is also the key to effective mediation – identify the points of concern and then deal with them one by one, openly and honestly.

When the issue concerned is a matter of opinion rather than of fact, things may be more complicated. However, the same principles still apply – identify the point for discussion and state your view clearly, however contentious. If the point for discussion is part of the agenda of a meeting and an immediate decision is going to be needed, it is sometimes a good idea to discuss the matter in advance with some of your colleagues. It is not always wise to make decisions on the spur of the moment, particularly if you are unsure of the views of the others involved in decision-making. A preliminary discussion will help make others aware of your point of view, and vice versa, so that any conflict can be identified and discussed. It is then more likely that you will be able to persuade a group to come around to your way of thinking. At all times, avoid stating your views rudely or too forcefully, just speak directly – the key difference between assertiveness and aggressiveness.

Effective clinical teams should, of course, put patients first, and have a number of key characteristics (Table 5). Successful teams should be able to demonstrate:

- purpose and value, including evidence of leadership, well-defined values, standards, functions and responsibilities, and clear strategic direction

- performance, including evidence of competent management, good systems, good performance records, effective internal performance monitoring, feedback and regular appraisal; in addition, all team members should accept responsibility for their own and each other's performance
- consistency, including evidence of thoroughness and a systematic approach to patient care and safety
- effectiveness and efficiency, including evidence of thorough medical and clinical audit
- a chain of responsibility, including evidence that the responsibilities of each of the team members are well defined and understood
- openness, such as transparency to others, evidence of comparative external review and performance measures that can be easily understood by those outside the team
- overall acceptability, including evidence that the overall performance and results achieved by the team inspire the trust and confidence of patients, employers and professional colleagues.

Table 5

Characteristics of successful teams

- Clear, shared objectives
- Good communication
- Supportive behaviour
- Trust
- Constructive criticism
- Shared workload
- Cooperation
- Balanced roles
- Decisions made by consensus
- Effective leadership
- Appropriate rewards

Leadership skills

Effective leadership skills are central to a motivated and fully functioning team that will dedicate its efforts towards the safe and efficient achievement of team goals. It is important to distinguish between leadership, which is acquired, and authority, which is assigned. As a team leader, you must influence the thoughts and behaviour of other team members through your own ideas and actions (Table 6), and your success will depend on the quality of your relationship with other team members. Coordinating team activities is a reciprocal process, and team members should feel that they have an integral role in the achievement of joint objectives.

As team leader, you must have a clear idea of the objective and must allocate tasks to team members according to their abilities and workload. An initial discussion will establish communication and ensure the support and participation of all team members. It will also provide an opportunity for other team members to contribute their views and ideas, and for any areas of contention to be resolved.

Being a good trainer

The most important aspect of being a good trainer is to interact with your trainees and encourage them to respond honestly and openly without fear of recrimination. Most trainers are very busy doctors, and training is yet another pressure on their time. It is very easy to allow trainees to settle into a new job, and possibly a new hospital, and for you to be only vaguely aware of their performance except when they are actually in your presence. Your very activity may prevent them from talking to you because they don't wish to interrupt or appear rude. A trainee may leave while you may have been only subconsciously aware that he or she was trying to approach you during the time with you. Positive action is required to prevent this from happening. Take time to greet each new trainee and arrange to meet when you have sufficient time – at least half an hour – to discuss adequately their past, the present attachment and their future. Set aside some time about halfway through the attachment to assess your trainee's progress, and then again to discuss their performance at the end of the attachment. Obviously, informal discussion during the attachment is valuable, but it is often impromptu and of ill-

Table 6

Leadership skills: attributes of good practice

Authority and assertiveness
- Take initiative to ensure team involvement
- If necessary, take command of situation and advocate own position
- Consider suggestions of others
- Motivate team through appreciation and provide coaching when necessary

Provision and maintenance of standards
- Adopt standard protocols and ensure team compliance
- Intervene if team performance deviates from standards
- Justify deviations from standard procedures when necessary following consultation with team
- Demonstrate the intention to achieve the highest possible standard under prevailing conditions

Planning and coordination
- Encourage team participation in planning and task completion
- Ensure that the plan is clearly stated, together with the goals and boundaries for task completion
- Change plan if necessary after consultation with team

Management of workload
- Allocate tasks to team members, and check and correct as appropriate
- Prioritize secondary operational tasks to retain sufficient resources for primary objectives
- Allow sufficient time to complete tasks
- In an emergency, offload: delegate those tasks that can be safely accomplished by junior team members (even if they will perform these tasks less well than more senior colleagues) in order to free more experienced team members to consider wider issues and to supervise the effort of the whole team
- Appreciate and allow for performance degradation due to stress or fatigue

continued...

Table 6 (continued)
Leadership skills: attributes of good practice

Improvements
- Review your own performance candidly and that of others sensitively
- Consider measures for improvement
- Note system failures and draw these to the attention of the management, with constructive suggestions if appropriate

defined duration, so that matters cannot always be dealt with properly. The fact that time has formally been set aside does not mean that these discussions need to be formal, but they should be taken seriously. In addition, formal appraisals should be undertaken, as discussed previously; informal discussion and formal appraisal can be grouped together three times a year so long as sufficient time is allowed for both.

You must be aware of your trainee's needs, both overall and in relation to his or her particular stage of training. You should be aware of what is involved and able to answer questions about the organizational aspects of training, as well as helping with clinical development. If you do not answer a trainee's questions, who will? In any specialty in which procedures must be learned it is essential that these procedures are taught. It is easy to excuse doing something yourself rather than allowing your trainee to do it on the grounds that you yourself are able to do it more quickly and to a higher standard. Supervising your trainee may take longer and the procedure may not be done quite as well as you would like, but often the end result is just as satisfactory and is a far more beneficial experience for the trainee. Patience in such situations is not only a virtue, but also a necessity!

Being a successful trainer is an integral part of being a successful doctor. Your role as a supportive, inspirational role model is vital to produce motivation for the successful doctors of the future. Don't fall into

> if **you do not answer** a trainee's questions, **who will?**

the trap of negativity towards change. This will only erode your own credibility and demoralize your team.

Learning from criticism

An important component of success is learning to cope with both criticism and failure. No-one is consistently successful. Indeed, Winston Churchill regarded success as 'the ability to go from failure to failure without losing your enthusiasm'.

In general, doctors do not take criticism well; however, failure obliges self-criticism and change. Constructive criticism can be a tool in creating future success. Doctors are currently subject to more criticism than ever before, as a result of social changes and increased access to information. Patients no longer consider doctors to be omniscient; they have high

criticism is a **gift**

expectations and are not afraid to complain if things do not go according to plan.

Patients who complain about their care or treatment have a right to a prompt and appropriate response. As a doctor, you have a professional responsibility to deal with complaints constructively and honestly. You must also comply with any complaints procedure that applies to your work. Never allow a patient's complaint to prejudice the care or treatment you arrange for that individual.

Learning to accept criticism positively and live with your failures – patients who cannot be saved, research that does not reveal a significant result and so on – early on in your career will stand you in good stead. Criticism is a gift; use the information provided constructively to make you and your team better doctors and more balanced people as a whole.

Further reading and resources

Clay B. Flexible training – what are the opportunities? [career focus]. *BMJ* 1998; 316(classified section 23 May):2–3.

Cooper CL. *Handbook of Stress Medicine and Health.* Boca Raton: CRC Press, 2005.

Donald A. Effective teaching [career focus]. *BMJ* 1998;317(classified section 18 July): 2–3.

Drife JO. Be interviewed. In: *How To Do It.* 2nd edn, vol 2. London: BMJ, 1998.

Gatrell J, White A. *Medical Student to Medical Director, A Development Strategy for Doctors.* Bristol: NHS Training Division, 1995.

General Medical Council. *The New Doctor.* London: GMC, 1997.

Gray C. Time management [career focus]. *BMJ* 1998;316(classified section 4 April):2–3.

Hall R. *Success.* London: Pearson Education, 2005.

Hardern R. Starting a new consultant post [career focus]. *BMJ* 1998;317(classified section 17 October):2–3.

Harris D, Peyton R, Walker M. Teaching in different situations. In: *Training the Trainers: Learning and Teaching.* London: Royal College of Surgeons, 1996.

Hobbs S. Learning from complaints. In: Lugon M, Secker-Walker J, eds. *Advancing clinical governance.* London: Royal Society of Medicine Press, 2001.

Leigh A, Maynard M. *Leading your Team.* London: Nicholas Brearley Publishing, 2002.

Morris S, Willcocks G, Knasel E. *How to lead a winning team.* London: Pearson Education, 2000.

Prosser S. *Effective People.* Oxford: Radcliffe Publishing, 2005.

Quick TL. *Successful Team Building.* New York: Amacom, 1992.

The Department of Health. *The New NHS. Modern. Dependable. A National Framework for Assessing Performance.* London: DH, 1998.
http://www.archive.official-documents.co.uk/document/doh/newnhs/contents.htm

Sharif K, Afnan M. Quality control in postgraduate training [career focus]. *BMJ* 1998;316(classified section 9 May):2–3.

making your name in private practice

'Never go to a doctor whose office plants have died'
Erma Bombeck (1927–1996)

The freedom of patients to choose private practice and for doctors to work independently alongside the NHS is enshrined in the 1946 National Health Service Act. Unlike the NHS, where any improvement or development has to be laboriously agreed with committees, colleagues and managers, in private practice you can manage your own time, build your own team, set your own strategic agenda and create an independent working environment geared towards business-like efficiency and financial success.

Quite apart from the fact that private practice is likely to enhance your income, it also provides important opportunities for a doctor's personal and clinical development, as well as the chance to hone his or her business skills. Additional attractions include a pleasant working environment, more time to spend with each individual patient and the opportunity to investigate and deal with underlying problems rapidly, efficiently and effectively.

> in **private practice** you can **manage** your **own time**

The formative stages

From the time that you take up your consultant post, you are entitled to establish a private practice, provided that this does not interfere with your sessional commitments within the NHS. These will have been agreed at the time of your appointment as part of your job plan, but can be renegotiated at a later date, usually with the chief executive and medical director of your hospital.

Traditionally, doctors have been reluctant to discuss private practice openly, and this has made the business of setting up more difficult. In fact, the best approach is to be frank and honest about your intentions, and discuss the key issues with your colleagues. Although you may be concerned that they will resent the competition ('another mouth to feed'), you will find that most colleagues will wish you as much success in this arena as they do in your NHS role. They would not have appointed you initially if they did not think you worthy of success!

Don't be afraid to ask your colleagues for advice about the best way to set up a private practice. Listen carefully to what they have to say, seek a second or even third opinion and then draw your own conclusions.

Before you begin, be certain that you have the time, energy and expertise to provide the highest level of care (Table 7).

Table 7
Provision of care

As in NHS practice, when working independently you must:

- Always work within the limits of your competence
- Provide effective treatments based on the best available evidence as defined by NICE
- Respect a patient's right to a second opinion
- Keep clear, accurate and legible records, reporting the relevant clinical findings, the decisions made and the information provided to patients, and any drugs prescribed or any investigation or treatment
- Be readily accessible when on duty and ensure that you are covered when you are not
- Consult and take advice from colleagues when appropriate

Adapted from General Medical Council. *Good Medical Practice* London: GMC, 2006.
http://www.gmc-uk.org/guidance/good_medical_practice/index.asp

---

Getting started

There are a number of ways to get started in private practice. You can:
- take sessions in a private hospital
- start a private practice in your own home
- rent your own dedicated rooms.

Each of these initiatives has strengths, weaknesses, opportunities and threats (SWOT). Think through your own SWOT analysis.

Taking the plunge in this way can be nail-biting stuff, but bear in mind that any new small business feels financially perilous for the first few months. Ultimately, long-term strategic thinking, with an element of initial risk-taking, is more likely to reap better rewards. However, it is possible to compromise by initially sharing rooms with a colleague – bearing in mind that many say one should choose one's consultant colleague more carefully than one's spouse!

> choose a **colleague** more carefully than a **spouse**

Private hospital sessions

Private hospital sessions are the cheapest and easiest option. This is usually a good way to start because you have the added advantage of working within a pleasant environment, with trained nursing staff and all the facilities you require for investigation of your patients. When you begin to work at a private hospital, they will often undertake a mailing on your behalf to inform referring GPs of your availability for consultations. In return, the hospital will usually charge you for the use of the facilities.

To get started, you should speak to the chief executive of your local private hospital and apply for admitting rights, which are usually granted by the medical advisory committee. The private hospital concerned will probably require references; your consultant colleagues may provide these, but it is always courteous to ask if they are willing to be referees before proposing them.

The drawback of private hospital sessions is that you do not have your personal office space and belongings around you, and sometimes the facilities are not much superior to those of the NHS.

Practising from home

Setting up in your own home is the time-honoured way to undertake private practice. Your home will need to be appropriate and the implications carefully considered in detail. You will also need to ensure that your consulting rooms are kept clean and tidy!

Running a business from home can have tax implications and may render you liable to capital gains tax on your house. Before deciding on this option, you should discuss your plans in some detail with your accountant (see Finance, pages 137–148) and your partner.

Renting your own rooms

Renting your own room is the most expensive option by far. However, it has the advantage that you will be available to see patients whenever you wish, and can have a secretary dedicated to taking calls and making appointments. Your own room becomes an extension of yourself. Personal effects, such as family photographs and degree certificates, in your office will provide your patients with important visual clues about you. This insight should encourage patients to form a favourable opinion of you and make them feel more comfortable about choosing you to look after them.

Staff

No man is an island, and in private practice, just as in the NHS, a calm, professional, efficient and effective team approach is needed. Your team is only as strong as its weakest link, and any human resources problems should be addressed, not ignored.

Most importantly, appoint a dedicated, competent secretary. The telephone needs to be manned for referrals from 9 a.m. to 5 p.m., and your secretary should be personable, intelligent and on the ball. Aim to employ someone with a positive attitude, and provide orientation and ongoing training. Strive to demonstrate the qualities that you expect of your secretary yourself. Avoid, for example, rolling your eyes to the ceiling when dealing with a difficult patient, or criticizing demanding relatives to your secretary. Although some people seem to enjoy it, negativity is rather contagious. It can permeate relationships with patients and staff alike, and may impair the overall performance of your practice. Some people fall into this pattern without realizing it. It helps to imagine creating a chart for yourself and checking how many positive and negative statements you make in one hour. How would you like to have yourself as a doctor, boss, spouse or friend?

Although your secretary is your most important team member (and one who has the power to make or break your practice), other team members each have an essential part to play.

- Is the receptionist welcoming and polite?
- If investigations are needed, are they completed in a well-organized, dignified and efficient manner?
- Are the results always accessible; can they be communicated to the patient?
- If a patient needs to be admitted, are the hospital staff cheerful, friendly and competent, and aware of the reason for admission?
- Finally, if the patient leaves a message with your secretary, do you always reply promptly, politely, effectively and professionally?

Working with colleagues

A weakness of private practice is the tendency for doctors to work alone. In fact, as in the NHS, teamwork is vital. If you are a surgeon, your key partner is your anaesthetist and it is important that you both work in harmony. For example, do you both provide the same information to patients? Do you both provide adequate pre- and postoperative patient review? Also, your partner's fee schedule should be compatible with yours.

Arranging cover

Another important consideration is the provision of medical cover when you are unavailable. Many private hospitals are introducing on-call rotas for consultants to ensure that there is always a consultant available to deal with unexpected emergencies. Remember, you must be satisfied that, when you are off duty or on holiday, suitable arrangements are made to cover your own patients' medical care. These arrangements should include effective handover procedures and clear communication (ideally written) between the doctors concerned. Be sure that the individual who is standing in for you has the experience, knowledge and skills to deal with the cases for which he or she will be responsible.

There is a growing trend for private practitioners to work in teams (Table 8). For example, four orthopaedic surgeons, experienced in different areas, might practise on a rota basis, referring patients within the team to the appropriate expert. This type of private group practice is likely to become more prevalent in the future and, currently, there is much discussion about doctors operating in 'chambers' in a similar manner to barristers. Such a move has considerable advantages in terms of sharing expenses, facilities, marketing and on-call commitments (Table 9). Critically for the venture, it should offer a better level of service for patients. However, choose your partners carefully before engaging in such an enterprise, as it is not unheard of for business partners to fall out!

Marketing your practice

In the UK, most patients gain access to a specialist via their GP. Therefore, marketing your practice largely depends on making referring physicians aware of your presence. In marketing, it is accepted that the average business never hears from 96% of its happy customers. However, unhappy

---

Table 8
Models for group private practice

- An informal group sharing premises, but retaining their own financial arrangements, including tax and accountancy matters
- In true partnership, as defined by the Partnership Act (1890), where members are responsible for each other's debts
- In a limited liability company with members owning shares, which offers significant tax advantages

---

Table 9

Models for consultants working together as an independent team

Informal group
- Share premises, but retain financial arrangements
- Some advantages, but no real financial gains

True partnership
- As defined by the 1890 Partnership Act, members are responsible for each other's debts
- Partnerships are risky and members have to trust each other implicitly

Limited liability company
- Members, and possibly other people, own shares
- Lower financial risk, but less favourable tax position when profits withdrawn

Limited liability partnership
- A new, and largely untried, model, which only became legal in 2001
- Combines the tax advantages of a partnership with the liability protection of a limited company

---

customers voice their concerns to, on average, nine or ten people – among them, in your case, undoubtedly the referring GP! Customers whose complaints are resolved tell, on average, only five people, and some of what they say may be positive.

To be successful, you should be able to offer expertise and technology that will allow you to diagnose and resolve patients' problems speedily and accurately. Other factors influencing whether patients are referred to you or to someone else include ease and speed of access to you, efficiency of feedback and whether or not patients are satisfied with their overall management and outcome.

Interaction with GPs can be achieved in a number of ways. Doctors starting out in private practice can send a mailing to all GPs in the area. If you move premises subsequently, another mailing is appropriate. Rules concerning advertising have recently been relaxed by the GMC, but it is still wise to be cautious about direct marketing to referring doctors. It is certainly inappropriate to criticize or denigrate a colleague or to claim that you offer a better service than a competitor, but a statement about your specific expertise, availability and how you can be contacted is acceptable, provided that it is factual and verifiable. In most parts of the UK, GPs will not refer private patients to you unless you and your team deliver a good service to their NHS patients.

GPs will **not refer** private patients **unless** you deliver a **good** service to their **NHS patients**

Regular contact with your referral sources is invaluable. Each letter you write to a GP serves to remind him or her of your practice. Articles you may write for journals read extensively by GPs, such as the *BMJ*, *Practitioner*, *Update* and *Pulse*, are indirect but valuable methods of marketing yourself or your unit ethically and enhancing your reputation. Presentations to GPs in postgraduate centres, where direct contact with your referring doctor can also be made in workshops and during the meal, are similarly useful. You may also meet and network with GPs at social events.

Direct marketing to patients is less important in the UK than in the USA because, in the UK, most patients are referred by their GPs and insurance companies are often reluctant to pay for those who are not. However, brochures for your patients with information about your practice are valuable. They should include the advice that patients cannot usually be seen without a referral from a GP. They should be well written and designed, as well as informative, presenting accurate information about you and a list of charges that the patient can expect. The Healthcare Commission now expect each private practitioner to produce a patient's guide. Although many doctors are reluctant to be up-front about their charges, patients almost always prefer them to be, as it allows them to clarify the extent of their cover with their insurer and relieves them of uncertainty about their liability. Approximately 20% of all private patients are uninsured and cover their own costs. A fixed-price package eases concern about unlimited liability for such patients. Draft brochures can be tested on your patients before the final version is produced. Ask questions such as 'If you could change one thing about this pamphlet, what would it be?'

Another way to improve your practice is to conduct patient surveys after treatment, assessing every stage in the service delivery. Assess satisfaction at each point of patient contact:

- original phone calls
- first consultation
- investigations
- treatment visits
- follow-up queries.

Ask, for example, 'How important is X to your overall satisfaction? And how well did we meet your expectations at Y?' Ensure that this exercise is meaningful – be prepared to act on the results of your survey.

Dealing with private patients

Success in private practice relies not only on referral from GPs, but also on recommendations from other patients. The quality of service that you offer is critical if word is to get around that you are the person to see for a certain problem. Of course, as with NHS patients, the following important principles apply:

- listen to patients and respect their views
- always treat patients professionally and considerately
- respect patients' privacy and dignity
- treat information about patients as strictly confidential
- give patients the advice they ask for or need about their condition, its treatment and prognosis.

Put yourself in the position of a patient who is worried about a symptom or condition and decides to call your practice to make an appointment.

- How many times does the telephone ring before it is answered?
- How polite and efficient is your secretary?
- What is the earliest appointment you can offer?

When the patient walks into your office, they will make a rapid judgement about whether they feel confident to have you as their doctor. Although this judgement will be made on much the same basis as that made by NHS patients, your patients will be very aware that they are paying for their consultations, and thus may have higher expectations.

A number of factors will influence how comfortable patients feel about you:

- your reputation as a caring and successful doctor, which goes before you and strongly influences patients' opinions
- the way you communicate to patients that you care about their problems and that you have the expertise to diagnose and treat those problems
- your physical environment, as patients will inevitably judge you by the setting they find you in
- your expertise in managing the patient's problem.

Your reputation is acquired only by the cumulative impact of a series of satisfied patients and good outcomes. For this and other reasons, it is critical that you do not over-extend yourself in private practice. One serious complication and its consequences can undo years of good results. In medicine, unnecessary risk-taking is hazardous and best avoided!

Financial dealings

It is crucial that you and everyone in your team are open and honest about any financial arrangements with patients. In particular:

- you must inform patients about your fees and charges, whenever possible before asking their consent for treatment
- you must not exploit patients' vulnerability or lack of medical knowledge when making charges for treatment or services
- you must not put pressure on patients or families to make donations to other people or organizations
- you must tell patients if any part of the fee goes to another healthcare professional.

Using the latest technology

Private practice lends itself to the use of the latest office technology. A number of user-friendly patient database systems are available. With the advent of scanners, it is possible to run a near-paperless office, creating a 'high-tech' image that is generally appreciated by patients. It is essential that every result or letter is scanned in as soon as it arrives; methodical and frequent backing up of files is mandatory. It is necessary, however, to retain a paper record for medicolegal purposes for at least 10 years. If your patients' files are wholly on computer, keeping paper records in chronological day files rather than in duplicate patient files will save hours of laborious sorting. Although a computer on your desk may convey the correct image, beware of being glued to your screen, and thereby losing eye contact with your patient. Information technology is likely to change the way medicine is practised over the next few years. Information about the NHS Care Records Service, which is currently under construction, is available at http://www.connectingforhealth.nhs.uk/clinicians.

Developing your own website is now an important component of the marketing of private practice. As with your brochure, this should be written in easy-to-read, plain English, and should set out the nature of your expertise. Some background information on the main conditions that you treat can be helpful, but these are often best supplied via links to larger, reputable, often US-based websites. UK charity sites are also useful to link to and may increase the number of hits on your site.

Using new technologies in the treatment of your patients can also be a way of boosting private practice. Minimally invasive devices, such as lasers and robots, have a tremendous appeal to patients and are often marketed on your behalf by the manufacturer and installed in private hospitals at their expense. Unfortunately, the results do not always live up to the initial hype. Moreover, your long-term credibility depends on you backing winners, so beware of espousing too avidly a new treatment method that later turns out to be a dead donkey!

Dealing with insurance companies

Health insurers can be like any other insurer – some seem to offer comprehensive cover until you make a claim, when you may find that the small print precludes that particular eventuality! Helping your patients through the maze of procedures involved in health insurance is an integral part of private practice.

When discussing health insurance with a patient, you must make it clear that they enter into a contract with you. Strictly speaking, the issue of whether the patient's insurance company will cover the cost of your fees is between the patient and their insurer. Patients should call the company's helpdesk to check that their consultations, investigations and inpatient procedures are covered. In practice, however, if you want to be reimbursed for your time and effort, you or a member of your team will need to facilitate the process of dealing with the insurance company.

Most private insurers reimburse only for acute rather than chronic illness. Many require a claim form to be completed, on which the date of onset of the condition and the date of referral are usually requested. Learn to use the OPCS procedure codes to classify diagnosis and treatment. Many companies also ask for the estimated waiting time for an NHS consultation for the patient's condition. You should answer this question candidly and to the best of your knowledge.

Avoiding the pitfalls

Never stray outside your own specialist area, however tempting it is to try to help out the patient by doing so. If problems occur, you must have the skills to deal with them. If you are dabbling in another specialty, this expertise will probably be lacking.

A second potential pitfall lies in the way in which you deal with complaints or complications that fall within your disease area. Be apologetic, honest and straightforward with patients and take the time to explain exactly what the problem is, what the short- and long-term problems are, and what you intend to do about it. If a second opinion or some specific expertise is needed, arrange for a senior colleague or a senior specialist in the relevant area to see the patient. Document all stages of the process clearly and accurately, and keep all parties fully informed. You should not withhold any relevant information. Do not be afraid to contact your medical defence union for advice – this is what you are paying (substantial amounts) for. If complications do occur, remember to exercise great sensitivity when submitting your bill. Receipt of an invoice after a long and protracted illness can be the final straw that persuades an unhappy patient to contact a solicitor!

In some specialties, such as dermatology and obstetrics and gynaecology, it may be appropriate to perform minor procedures in your rooms rather than in the operating theatre. If you do so, remember that the same strict rules that are enforced in the NHS regarding sterility and the disposal of human waste and sharp objects, such as needles and scalpels, are applicable to private practice and must be adhered to scrupulously. If you practise solely in the private sector, you must be registered with the Healthcare Commission; failure to register is an offence against the Care Standards Act 2000 part II section 11(1). Nowadays, if you are a fully independent practitioner or larger private operation, you can anticipate an inspection by the Healthcare Commission. After a detailed inspection they will publish the results of their visit on their website, warts and all. Be aware that they have the power to close down practices that do not meet their exacting standards.

Remember, in private practice, as in NHS medicine, you must not:

- use your position to establish improper personal relationships with patients or their close relatives
- improperly disclose or misuse confidential information about patients
- give, or recommend, to patients an investigation or treatment that you know is not in their best interest
- permit anyone who is not registered with the GMC to carry out tasks that require the training, knowledge and skills of a doctor – for example, to prescribe drugs or undertake procedures in the operating theatre.

Don't forget, though, that when you get it right private practice can be immensely satisfying and produce the highest standard of personalized and innovative patient care.

Further reading and resources

General Medical Council. *Good Medical Practice* London: GMC, 2006.
http://www.gmc-uk.org/guidance/good_medical_practice/index.asp

National Institute for Health and Clinical Excellence (NICE)
http://www.nice.org.uk

effective communication

'Only connect'
Howards End, EM Forster (1910)

Clear, concise and effective communication is essential in all aspects of medicine. To be a successful doctor, you must develop the ability to establish a rapid rapport, first and foremost with patients, but also with colleagues, managers and other healthcare professionals. Good communication depends not only on content but also on delivery. Both must be adjusted according to the audience and the setting. The skilful educator (as opposed to lecturer) connects with an audience, addressing issues that are relevant and important to them, as well as supplying new information in a thought-provoking way.

Talking to your patients

Talking to patients is not always easy, particularly in the setting of the busy clinic or the wards. There are, however, a number of golden rules that, if followed, will help you to do this effectively.

As a patient enters your office or cubicle, stand up and shake their hand. Even better, go and collect your patient from the waiting room. Make a 'connection' by listening attentively and avoid interrupting – one study suggested that most doctors interrupt within 19 seconds of the interview commencing! Apologize for any delay, establish eye contact and always try to be concerned, interested and focussed (Table 10). Ensure that you allow yourself sufficient time to glean all the salient points of the case and, when appropriate, perform a gentle and professional physical examination. You should give your opinion emphatically, but in a friendly and sympathetic way. Throughout the consultation take care to speak clearly and concisely, avoiding medical jargon, acronyms and technical terms. Listen to your patient, don't pontificate or patronize. Ensure, whenever practical, that arrangements are made to meet patients' language and communication needs.

Table 10

Communicating with patients

- Listen to patients, ask for and respect their views about their health and respond to their concerns and preferences
- Share with patients, in a way that they can understand, the information they want or need to know about their condition, its likely progression and the treatment options open to them, including the associated risks and uncertainties
- Respond promptly to patients' questions and keep them informed about the progress of their care
- Make sure that patients are informed about how information is shared within teams and among those who will be providing their care, and with the patient's relatives and friends

When it comes to investigation and treatment, discuss the pros and cons of each option with your patient. Listen to your patients' opinions; they are more likely to comply with a treatment plan into which they have had some input. Nowadays, the concept of a doctor–patient partnership has replaced the paternalism of old. Patients want to be talked to, not at! Important messages still need to be repeated and reinforced several times because stressed and anxious patients may absorb only a fraction of what they are told. It may be helpful for patients if you write down the key points or draw a quick sketch for them to take away.

patients want to be talked to, not at

Never give the impression that you are in a hurry. Be sure to switch off your mobile phone and do not have phone calls put through to you during a consultation. You do not want your patient to think someone else's time is more important to you than theirs.

Remain focussed on the case throughout the consultation; at the end, summarize the agreed treatment plan, stand up and escort your patient to the door and shake hands again, maintaining eye contact and reinforcing key messages. Make sure that the follow-up arrangements are understood. If possible, give your patient literature that provides relevant and understandable, independent information about their condition. Tell patients about websites and support groups, and make sure contact details and written material are available. Make it clear that you are focussed on their problem and that you care.

The internet: breakthrough or breakdown?

When prescribed a new treatment or when newly diagnosed with a disease, many patients crave information, and they now have access to more information regarding their conditions and treatments than ever before, but much of it is unchecked or unreliable, some of it is promotional and it is seldom evidence-based. We have all been confronted with patients bearing reams and reams of printouts, quite possibly from websites based outside the European Union and governed by legislation very different from that in the UK. For example, in the USA prescription-only medicines can be promoted directly to patients, while this is illegal within the European Union. Knowledge that the patient has gained from less authoritative sources may be used to challenge your position and undermine the doctor–patient relationship, which will take time and patience to re-establish.

The internet is a powerful tool that is already proving invaluable. There is no question that it is changing all our lives, and the profession needs to embrace it rather than be left behind. Since patients expect their doctor to be better informed than themselves, the medical information freely available through the internet is likely to pose an increasing challenge, and one that you must address by keeping scrupulously up to date.

Breaking bad news

How bad news should be conveyed to patients and relatives is seldom discussed seriously by doctors. As malignancies, accidents and other potentially fatal conditions are commonplace, you may find yourself in the position of delivering bad news. A patient will never forget the moment he or she receives the diagnosis of a terminal illness. Historically, doctors have shied away from telling their patients the truth: in 1672, the

French physician Samuel de Sobière considered the idea, but discounted it on the grounds that it might seriously jeopardize his medical practice!

In 1961, a landmark paper by Oken revealed that 90% of surgeons in the USA would not routinely discuss a diagnosis of cancer with their patients. Subsequent studies, however, showed that a growing number of patients desperately wanted to know about and understand their diagnosis. Attitudes in this respect have adapted gradually, particularly in the USA, such that a repeat survey almost 20 years after the original showed that US physicians had completely reversed their attitudes, with more than 90% saying they would tell a patient if they had cancer. This change has not necessarily been accomplished as rapidly in other parts of the world: in the UK, a survey of family physicians and hospital consultants in the early 1980s showed that 75% and 56%, respectively, still did not routinely tell their patients the truth about a cancer diagnosis.

It is not difficult to understand the main reasons why clinicians wish to avoid sharing bad news with their patients. It can be a harrowing experience to be the messenger of doom, and subsequently have to provide patients with the support they need while they absorb and grapple with the true nature of their illness and prognosis. Traditionally, clinicians have found two main justifications for keeping patients and their families in the dark. First, the facts may upset them. This is undoubtedly the case, but this line of reasoning is not acceptable to any other profession in which news may be bad, for example, stockbrokers or lawyers. Second, doctors, and sometimes close relatives, presume that patients do not really want to know. In fact, several studies have confirmed the opposite to be true. In a survey of 250 patients attending a cancer centre in Scotland, 79% wanted to know as much as possible about their disease and 96% specifically wanted to know if their disease was cancer. Almost all patients wanted to know their realistic chance of cure and to be given details about possible side-effects of treatment. They also wanted to decide who else should be told. All patients felt that family members should be informed provided that the patient had given permission, but nearly two-thirds felt that if the patient did not wish relatives to know, then the family should not be taken into confidence.

most **patients want** to **know** as much as possible **about their disease**

Sharing with your patient

How, then, should a caring physician break bad news to a patient newly diagnosed with a life-threatening condition? Not surprisingly, most doctors feel uneasy when in such a position, and perhaps anxiety about communication techniques underlies most arguments for not telling the patient the truth. Many of us have had little or no counselling training, and we are often pushed for time in our busy clinics. The difficulty is to convey the information sensitively and supportively, and in a way that the patient can understand (Table 11). You should not appear rushed. Many of our own patients have admitted that they understood hardly anything they were told in the traumatic interview when the bad news was broken: 'As soon as you said the word cancer, doctor, my mind went blank.' Try to find a quiet, private place, where interruptions are unlikely, to convey the news. Also, attempt to develop a connection with the patient and then offer to share the news with him or her, rather than simply blurting it out. It is important to counterbalance bad news with support and information.

Having a close relative in the consulting room means there is a second person to absorb the information, as well as to provide emotional support to the affected individual. Providing written information about the disease, which can be digested later when the patient has recovered from the initial impact of the news, is usually much appreciated. Easy-to-understand literature should be available, as patients often have a large number of questions. Ideally, specially trained nurses should be at hand to provide counselling and support for patients, both immediately upon disclosure of the diagnosis of a terminal illness and afterwards as the news gradually sinks in. Information on specific patient support groups can also be very helpful – many now have a valuable presence on the internet.

Supporting close relatives

The impact of cancer on a patient's partner is another important, but often neglected, area of concern. For example, the treatments used in prostate cancer commonly affect sexual function and these need to be discussed not only with the patient but also with his spouse. The consequences of loss of libido, erectile dysfunction and ejaculatory disturbances must be explained sympathetically to both partners. Failure to do so effectively may have a devastatingly negative impact on their

Table 11

A framework for breaking bad news

Preparation
- Familiarize yourself with all the information
- Have the case notes with you
- Ensure you have ample time
- Make sure that the environment is comfortable and private
- Avoid interruptions (bleeper, phone, BlackBerry™ etc)

Introductions
- Introduce yourself and any other staff
- Identify everyone else (i.e. relatives, friends) and address them formally

Knowledge
- Ascertain current understanding and thoughts
- Determine the patient's desired level of involvement in decision-making and treatment

Giving information
- Explain the situation honestly and sensitively
- Use plain English
- Use appropriate pacing and repetition
- Allow pauses and questions
- Be empathic, and don't be afraid to say 'sorry' or 'I don't know'
- Don't argue with or criticize colleagues
- Ensure that you address the patient's concerns
- Encourage questions
- Be honest about the options if treatment has to be deferred

Finally
- Plan a further meeting and/or 'leave the door open'
- Try to leave some hope
- Be alert to your own feelings and those of other staff; debriefing sessions may be valuable

relationship. Men, and older men in particular, diagnosed as suffering from cancer are particularly reliant on the social support that stems from intimate relationships, and withdrawal from sexual relationships may have severe consequences on both their quality of life and their overall health. Sympathetic, unhurried counselling of the couple about this aspect of their lives, as well as about treatment options and their possible side-effects, is therefore vital.

The essential skills

Learning how to break bad news sympathetically and effectively is a fundamental skill to acquire. Nowadays, there is no excuse for the clinician who simply does not want to perform this important part of the job. It is an essential part of a doctor's role and, with attention to detail, can be done well. It has wisely been said that, 'If the breaking of bad news is done badly, patients and their families may never forgive us; in contrast, if we get it right they will never forget us'. The challenge for clinicians everywhere is to improve and enhance this most important aspect of their communication skills.

Communicating with dying patients

Death doesn't always come to us as a friend, and in no other situation is good communication between doctors, patient and relatives more important, or potentially more fraught. Remember that, in a family, death is associated with all sorts of concomitant tensions. Not only are the relatives trying to deal with the demise of a loved one, but they may also be confronting other compromising issues, such as financial hardship, feelings of guilt or problematic family relationships.

One problem of which we should be acutely aware is the lack of public understanding about the way today's NHS functions. Many people have fond memories of how things were years ago – matrons, plenty of beds and access to the same doctor continually. However, things have changed. The level of emergency admissions means that patients are placed where a bed is available, often on wards nursed by staff not familiar with a particular patient's condition. This inevitably leads to fragmented communication. In addition, the reduction in junior doctors' hours makes it less likely that a familiar doctor will be available to talk to relatives.

Attitudes of the public have also changed. The assumption that the doctor is necessarily right has been undermined and there is a much greater reluctance to accept death as an inevitable outcome, no matter how old or how ill the patient.

The key to the problem is good communication. Lack of information makes people feel powerless, and powerlessness can lead to aggression. Doctors need to communicate effectively with all members of the medical team. Timely and appropriate information must be given to the patient and relatives in a friendly, professional and sympathetic manner. In the words of Dame Cicely Saunders, founder of the hospice movement, 'Remember, five minutes' conversation on a timely basis can save hours of work later on. It is not so much the quantity of time, but the quality of time that is critical.'

Communicating with colleagues and managers

To be successful as a doctor, you have to be perceived as such by your colleagues and managers – this is your 'reputation'. The way in which you communicate with them on clinical or academic matters is critical to the position in which they place you in their own mental hierarchy. It may seem obvious, but keep in mind that people prefer a friendly, affable, optimistic colleague to a taciturn, abrasive and pessimistic one, and are far more likely to relate to and support the former. A good tip is to be friendly to and treat with respect everyone you work with, from the chief executive to the ward cleaners. Remember that it is not an especially endearing characteristic to be sycophantic to those above you in the hierarchy and tyrannical to those below!

As doctors meet so many colleagues, first impressions are particularly important. Shaking hands, maintaining eye contact and remembering the name of a new acquaintance is very helpful. Sir Yehudi Menuhin, arguably the most successful musician of the 20th century, used to visit his music school only once or twice a year, but would always make an effort to speak to each and every pupil and recall their names and details. Remember that every corridor meeting or telephone conversation is a communication exercise. After meeting or talking to you, people will form an impression – good communication helps to make it a positive impression.

Dealing with the media

Dealing with the media is an increasingly important communication skill for the modern doctor and an excellent way of raising your own profile. The best way to acquire this is to attend a media skills course, at which you will be able to obtain some practical experience through radio and television interview role-play and subsequent post-mortem audiovisual analysis of your performance.

When dealing with the media, at all times think of the message you want to convey and the image you are trying to create – caring, composed and competent – and the one you are trying to avoid, that of being aloof, arrogant and defensive. On television, body language is critical in this respect. Look directly at the interviewer or camera. Try to appear relaxed. Avoid adopting defensive body positions and fiddling with your hands, nose or ears. Use gestures sparingly. Even raising a finger during a television interview can look like an exaggerated and aggressive gesture to the viewers. Avoid wearing white shirts or narrow striped ties during a TV recording session because of potential adverse camera effects. In radio interviews, keep your audience and message in mind at all times. Speak slowly and clearly, and avoid using medical jargon. To give yourself time to think, rephrase the question as the start to your answer. Avoid beginning with 'er...', which has been aptly described as 'the noise of thinking aloud'.

Remember that your best weapon is your clinical skill and experience. TV and radio journalists seldom attack doctors, although this is changing in the current, increasingly negative, climate. If you are criticized, respond positively – try to convey the message that medicine is not an easy business, but in spite of this the vast majority of cases go well. Keep your answers simple, short and straightforward. Before the interview, try to think of a catchy sound bite that encapsulates your message, and end the interview on a positive note.

Caution is needed when dealing with newspaper or magazine journalists. Beware making an impromptu remark that may be

good news does not sell newspapers

taken out of context and splashed across the front page. Remember that medicine is full of human-interest stories that the media love, and that good news does not sell newspapers. Above all, avoid breaching patient confidentiality or denigrating your colleagues, institution or the NHS publicly. Before accepting a call from a journalist, think very carefully about what you want to say and try to put a positive spin on the issue in question. For example, you might point out that although one healthy kidney was mistakenly removed recently at St Elsewhere's, some 7999 successful operations were performed in the same year across the UK.

Making oral presentations

Good presentations do not just happen – they are the result of careful planning and scrupulous preparation. Interesting and relevant content, clear delivery and a variety of visual and auditory techniques all contribute to an effective presentation. To borrow from Tolstoy's opening line in *Anna Karenina*: 'Good presentations are all alike; every bad presentation is bad in its own way.'

Developing the text

The spoken word needs to be much simpler and more straightforward than the written word. To make your message clear, remember the adage: 'Tell them what you are going to tell them, tell them, and then tell them what you have told them.' Use plain, simple English and try to illustrate your points with word pictures; many people will remember information that is told as a story or anecdote rather than dry facts or ideas.

Know and connect with your audience. Avoid the 'So what?' factor by asking yourself 'What is the audience hoping to get out of this talk?' At the same time, consider your message and how best to convey it. Make it clear very early on in the talk why your subject is relevant and exactly 'what's in it' for the attendees. Be clear about what you want the audience to take away with them. Also consider the setting – find out who or what will precede and follow your talk. Make sure that your presentation fits in with the overall theme.

It is crucial to be thoroughly prepared for your presentation.

- Research your topic and write one first draft, setting out all your ideas and facts.
- Work through this draft and underline the key points.

- Write these out on separate pieces of paper, and then go back to your first draft and find statements, facts or examples that corroborate your main points – use these sparingly.
- Your audience's time is precious – do not waste it with inappropriate, too detailed or irrelevant information.
- Use logical development; try to link one major point with the next.
- Mark the points that can be made more effectively with a slide or overhead.
- Stand back and ask yourself whether the message is relevant and clear, and what it will give the audience.

Preparing your delivery

However well prepared your text, it will not be appreciated unless it is delivered in a lively, enthusiastic fashion. Do not memorize your talk – you risk forgetting a segment and grinding to an embarrassing and seemingly eternal halt. If this happens at a major presentation, believe me, you will blush at the memory for a very long time! Learn the first two lines of your talk, and after that speak spontaneously and with energy. Write the key points on numbered cards. You will also have your slides or overheads as prompts, but get to know them intimately and avoid using them as a crutch by following them slavishly. Practise your talk four or five times. Do not just run through it silently – actually try to recreate the setting and speak your words out loud.

speak spontaneously and with **energy**

On the day, arrive early and check the facilities, such as slide-changing buttons, carefully before you ascend the podium. Think 'if it can go wrong, it will go wrong' and be prepared for exigencies. Finally, look after all equipment carefully; treat your computer leads as a sailor would his ropes!

Delivery

After your talk, people will leave not only with the information that you have supplied (if they have listened), but also with an impression of you. This stems not from what you say, but how you say it (Table 12). Body

Table 12

How to deliver your presentation effectively

- Dress comfortably but appropriately
- Try to stand squarely towards the audience, with legs slightly apart
- Make eye contact and do not ignore any section of the audience
- Have an arresting, confident opening
- Use appropriate hand gestures
- Do not talk to your slides
- Speak slowly, inflect your voice and enunciate each word
- Pause for emphasis, but speak in complete sentences
- Do not overuse the laser pointer (particularly if nerves produce a hand tremor!)
- Repeat important points
- Use concrete examples
- Convey enthusiasm
- Pose questions and give possible answers
- Explain the significance of points
- Summarize the talk
- Suggest what the audience should do with the information

language – your posture, stance and arm movements – is an important part of your image.

Avoid the monotonous delivery that sedates an audience so effectively! Smile and enthuse – if you are not interested in your subject, why should your audience be? Use voice inflection, pauses, tone and pace – speak slowly, loudly and deliberately. Do not talk to your slides as you will inevitably turn away from the audience and the microphone.

Humour is a powerful way to establish and maintain audience rapport. But making people laugh is not a matter of telling jokes. In general, avoid jokes unless you can deliver them with timing and congruence – a joke that falls flat stays down a long time, along with your talk. 'Fun' is not the same as 'funny'; often all you need to do to raise a smile and get the audience on your side is point out the odd or unusual aspects of something quite mundane.

Effective communication

Visual aids

Good slides or overheads add interest to your presentation and provide another medium for communicating your key messages. They allow an audience to focus on the salient points. However, unclear, crowded slides with spelling mistakes will do little to enhance your image and credibility. Follow the golden rules for effective visuals (Table 13) – 80% of what your audience remembers is what they see.

Table 13

Making the most of slides and overheads

- Each slide or overhead should have a specific purpose; limit each to one main idea
- Be accurate – mistakes on visuals stand out and force the speaker into an apologetic mode
- Aim for simplicity and conciseness – do not overload your slide with information
- Design slides so that the back row of your audience can see them clearly and understand them: print the slide at A4 size, lay it on the floor, stand on a chair next to it and see whether you can read it
- Use strong, bold sans serif typefaces and lower-case lettering for legibility
- Use ample spacing between lines, no more than seven words per line and a maximum of seven lines per slide
- Ensure axes and data lines on graphs are sufficiently bold to be clearly visible
- Minimize punctuation; use bullet points
- Use light-coloured text (ideally yellow or white) on a dark background
- Use a consistent style between slides – they can then be mixed for future presentations
- Summarize the 'take-home' messages on your final slide
- Develop a style that suits your personality

Always check the size of the room that you will be presenting in. Ensure that people at the back of the room will be able to read your slides, otherwise you risk losing their attention. Do not try to present too many slides – allow each slide to be shown long enough for everyone to read. As a guideline, a 15-minute presentation should be accompanied by no more than 15–20 slides. As each slide comes up, pause and then tell the audience what it says and what it means; this technique is known as 'clearing the visual'.

do not clutter the slides

Everyone now uses Microsoft PowerPoint™ software to make presentations directly from their own laptop or from a disk. These can be very effective and do project an image of someone who is able to work with technology. There are some pitfalls, however, because of the potential glitches associated with using any computer. Take time to learn how to use the software properly – there are many short courses and good manuals available.

be prepared to talk without slides

Do not clutter the slides or overuse the animation that PowerPoint allows – remember that in good communication less is more. Immediately before your presentation, ensure that computer and projector are working properly; you do not want to stand on the podium looking abject because your slides or video clips do not appear on the screen. If the system does crash, be prepared to talk without slides – the show must go on!

Handling questions

Question time can be nerve-racking, but it can also be fun and the highlight of your talk. Responding naturally and effectively to the audience is the best way to get them on your side. Try to avoid answering too quickly, or giving too detailed an answer. Repeat the question and then answer clearly and briefly, looking directly at the questioner. Do not let one questioner – particularly a dominant and aggressive one – monopolize your time. Instead, try to move on to another – with luck more positive – questioner. You can do this by pointing out that only one question is allowed from any member of the audience and turning away to a different part of the auditorium, although strictly speaking this is the chairman's responsibility. Use question time as an opportunity to repeat your message. Always end on a positive, 'high' note – many good presentations are spoilt by a lack of confidence when closing. Try not to rush from the podium, obviously

> always **end** on a
> **positive note**

relieved to have survived your ordeal; remove your lapel microphone, smile and return to your seat in the auditorium in a composed and professional manner.

Poster presentations

As the number of people attending international conferences continues to grow, posters are being used increasingly as a method of communicating research data to a wide audience. Posters are a very effective and flexible tool, allowing viewers to study information in as much or as little detail as they wish. Good preparation is essential; read any instructions carefully and adhere to them. Do not try to overload the poster with information. Ensure that the text is concise, simple and supported with appropriate graphics. Divide the content into the following sections:

- aims
- introduction
- methods
- results
- conclusions
- references.

Consider the design aspects of the poster. Make sure the text is large enough to be read at a short distance, and do not introduce too many different typefaces, as this will detract from the content. Use colour sparingly, considering the overall visual impact of the poster, while trying to make it both attractive and informative. If you have to present your poster, do so without slides, summarizing the key points of the work succinctly – it is not an opportunity to give a 7-minute lecture! Always be enthusiastic, confident, timely and professional.

Chairing small meetings and committees

The way in which you chair committees or meetings can greatly influence your peers' and colleagues' perception of you. By being prepared, you will develop a reputation for being a reliable, effective and stimulating chairman. Your role as chairman of a meeting is to manage:

- individual speakers
- the group
- yourself.

To do this effectively requires thorough planning; too many chairmen arrive at the last moment and try to wing it. This is a waste of time and is discourteous to all in attendance. Ideally, you should have studied and thought about the session in some detail, prepared relevant questions and, if possible, made arrangements to meet each speaker or participant before the session. By taking the following actions, you will ensure that every attendee gets the most from the meeting and that the meeting fulfils its objectives:

- circulate the agenda and talk to colleagues before the meeting; if possible, establish whether they are potential supporters or opposers of the scheme(s) you have in mind
- arrive early and start on time, make the necessary introductions, run through the agenda, but allow everybody to have their say
- be pleasant, but firm and direct; never show irritability, argue or make personal remarks about individuals – people tend not to forget them and may harbour a grudge for years afterwards
- always try to finish punctually, making a succinct and upbeat summary of the session, and thank each of the speakers and members of the group for their participation.

Chairing academic sessions

The success of an academic session depends not only on the quality of the science presented, but also on the way in which information is delivered. Consequently, being asked to chair an academic session should be considered a privilege, and is a role not to be undertaken lightly. As chairman, you will need to manage the session (and yourself) carefully. Therefore, you must set the guidelines for the session, facilitate the discussion and summarize the take-home messages in a simple, concise and relevant way. Before the meeting, you should:

- meet the speakers, stressing the importance of keeping to the allocated time and leaving sufficient time for questions
- agree a timing signal, and agree a procedure should the presentation over-run
- decide how questions will be handled
- agree a signal the speakers should use should they want the chairman to intervene.

Remember, you never have a second chance to make a first impression, and what you wear is fundamental to this. Dressing too casually will suggest that the meeting is not important, whereas smart clothing will project the correct image. You should also appear confident and professional, but remain calm and relaxed throughout the proceedings.

Establishing eye contact with both the speaker and audience will convey your interest and involvement in the session. When each talk is over, make eye contact with the speaker to put him at ease. Be careful not to display any form of body language that communicates a lack of interest to the audience – never fidget, fiddle or look bored!

Opening the session

Your objectives at the start of a session are to generate interest among, and engage the attention of, the audience, encouraging them to be receptive to the presentations. By introducing yourself and briefly mentioning your credentials for the job, you will begin to establish a rapport with the audience. Highlight the objective of the session and enthuse the audience by stating its relevance to them; describe how the session will be structured and how questions will be handled.

Handling questions effectively

Managing the questions session is perhaps one of the biggest challenges of chairmanship. Clearly, it is the responsibility of the speakers to respond to the questions, but as chairman you too should play an active role. When a talk finishes, thank the speaker and encourage the audience to provide their perspective. Calculate in advance how much time to allow for each question, and keep the discussion flowing to allow as many people as possible to participate. Make sure questioners state their names and institutions before asking their questions. If people with vested interests are present, such as employees of pharmaceutical companies, they should politely be asked to state their company and any potential conflict of interests. You should always have a question or two prepared in case there are none from the floor.

Although most are fairly straightforward, there are occasions when peripheral questions or rambling questioners distract from the objective of the session. Take control of the situation, perhaps suggesting that the questioner meet with the speaker after the session. Ensure that dominant personalities do not monopolize the proceedings (one way to do this is to insist on one question only from any member of the audience), and that those with the most to contribute have an opportunity to do so. If you are chairing a panel discussion, do not let the panel members dominate at the expense of audience participation. When all the questions have been asked or time has run out, do not let the session peter out – close it on a positive, forward-thinking note.

Publications

Before committing yourself to any writing or editing project, find out about the expected publication schedule. Proceed with the project only if you are confident that you will be able to give it the attention that it deserves throughout the duration of its production. An author who does not deliver or needs to be repeatedly chased makes life unpleasant for himself or herself as well as for editors and publishers. This will not win you friends or respect, and if word spreads that you are a 'non-deliverer', invitations to contribute to publications in the future will not be forthcoming.

Curriculum Vitae

Because doctors have to apply so many times for jobs, even in the new era of MMC, a high-impact CV is essential. John Middleton has written an excellent book on the subject, and the reader is referred to that text (Middleton J. *High-Impact CVs*. Oxford: Infinite Ideas, 2005). Make sure that you have a well-written, up-to-date CV on your laptop ready to e-mail within a day or so of a request to see it or at the sight of a job vacancy that interests you.

Writing

Writing is a skill, not a talent, and can be improved by practice and painstaking thought. Clarity is your goal, and it requires careful consideration and meticulous attention to detail. Although you may feel that there is a world of difference between writing an article for a peer-reviewed journal and becoming involved with writing for patients, the basic principles are the same (Table 14).

The most vital questions to ask yourself are 'Who are my readers?', 'What are their needs?' and 'What is my message?' Keep these in mind throughout the writing process.

Table 14
Effective writing

- Don't try to impress the reader with your expansive vocabulary; put that thesaurus down!
- Use as few words as possible without slipping into note form
- Use short words rather than long ones
- Use jargon and acronyms only when writing exclusively for fellow specialists
- Restrict sentences to 15–20 words, with only one idea per sentence or clause
- Use your words with accuracy and clarity
- Use bullet points rather than hiding lengthy lists in your text (they make text less visually daunting)
- Use different levels of headings (having checked the style of the publication, of course); like bullet points, they break up the text
- Avoid clichés like the plague!
- Check that any numbers (especially drug doses) and any statistics are correct
- Keep your reader and your message in mind at all times

Now, what is your brief? Are you writing a paper for submission to a journal, a poster or a chapter for a book, perhaps? Look at the guidelines carefully and, if possible, look at some samples of the type of work wanted. Do you need an introduction? How detailed should the discussion of your methods be? Can you include figures and tables, and if so, in what format? What level of referencing is required? Avoid thinking that you know what is wanted without checking. One of the problems that editors encounter is finding that authors have written what they want to write, rather than what they have been asked for.

The next step is to research the topic, and then put all your ideas, supporting facts and arguments down on paper. Start by drafting an outline. From there, it is not too difficult to organize your main points in order of importance, adding details to support each main point. At this stage, you are ready to write. Stick to the outline and start with the main ideas and their supporting details. Once this is done, revise the text and consider how well your message has been conveyed and whether the reader will be satisfied.

> you **are** what
> you **write**

Finally, enjoy watching the list of publications grow on your CV, PubMed and Medline, but remember that in hospital medicine you are what you write. Inflated publication claims, plagiarism and dual publication can easily be detected electronically these days.

Submitting to a journal

If you are submitting a paper to a peer-reviewed journal, you will have to deal effectively with reviewers' comments and will probably be expected to check page proofs (see page 93). If, for some reason, you find that you will not have the opportunity to check your submitted article before publication, scrutinize it closely before submission – pay particular attention to drug regimens and dosages, experimental data and the results of any calculations. Also, double-check the results of any other studies that you may have included in your introduction or discussion. Follow the instructions for submission of articles carefully, and always keep copies of everything that you send to the journal.

Working with a medical communications or public relations agency

Writing for a pharmaceutical-company-sponsored publication can be both lucrative and satisfying – publications are usually of the highest quality and it can be a thrill to see your name adorning such an attractive piece of work. However, your first encounter with this type of company may be something of a shock. You may be approached by either a product manager or other representative from a pharmaceutical company, or by an account manager or editor of the agency working on the pharmaceutical company's behalf. Before committing yourself to anything, you must make sure that you are completely clear about your role, the aim of the publication, how your name will be used, who has editorial control, how much work is involved and the schedule.

The type of project varies widely, but each publication has a role in marketing the company's drug or product. You may simply be asked to write a short article on your specialist subject, which will be very lightly edited, returned to you for approval and then published. Fine, but will the pharmaceutical company's logo be flashed across the cover? If you are uncomfortable with such an association, then steer clear of this type of work. (See *The Blue Guide: Advertising and Promotion of Medicines in the UK*, available from the Medicines and Healthcare products Regulatory Agency, http://www.mhra.gov.uk/.)

At the other end of the scale, you may be asked to put your name to a piece of work that has been drafted on your behalf. Be cautious about this – agree only if it reflects accurately your own convictions. This approach may seem favourable in terms of efficiency of time, but this is not always the case. Although you will save time at the outset, you must invest time checking the article thoroughly – after all, it will be carrying your name. Many experts find that, having looked through a drafted article, they prefer to rewrite most of it anyway.

Leaving ghost-writing to one side, the first time that you receive an edited version of something that you have written for an agency, you may think that there has been some sort of mistake. The article returned to you may only bear a passing resemblance to the one that you submitted! The role of editing in agency circles is very different from that for journals. As well as ensuring that your article reads well and is appropriate for the anticipated audience, the agency editor must make sure that the text fits the space allocated exactly, meets the marketing brief of the client and conforms to the house style of either the agency or the client company. House-style rules apply to wording, phraseology and the layout of articles. They may seem petty, but are necessary in publishing circles, as they enforce some sort of standardization on a company's products. You will probably never notice the effects of house styling, but if you find that something you have written has been changed consistently but for no obvious reason (e.g. if each time 'especially' appeared in your manuscript, it has been changed to 'particularly'), it is likely to be the result of editing into house style.

So, you have the edited version of your article in your hand. The best approach is to try to read the article as if it was a completely new piece of work. Does it make sense? Is it accurate? Does it flow well? You may think that your original version was better, but if you can answer 'yes' to the preceding questions, there is probably little reason to make a fuss. However, on occasion you may find that the article no longer makes sense or you will spot inaccuracies that have been introduced. Most editors have science degrees, many have PhDs, but few have specialist medical knowledge. Their work is based on your original article, so if they have completely misinterpreted something then perhaps it was not clear in the first place.

Good editors know when they are confused and will incorporate queries into the text for you to answer. Always answer these as clearly as possible, no matter how obvious the answer may appear to you. If you have real concerns about your article, talk to your editor and try to reach a compromise. If you are still unhappy, contact the account manager and suggest that another editor look at what has been done. If you still cannot reach a compromise, investigate the ease with which you can withdraw from the project; this will depend on any agreement you have made with either the agency or the pharmaceutical company.

Mark your comments clearly on to the manuscript using blue ink – your comments will be visible and the pages will also photocopy well. Print or use capitals if your handwriting is at all unclear. Using standard proof-correction marks in the margin will help the editor to interpret your amendments accurately (see, for example, http://www.ideography.co.uk/proof/proofmarks.pdf). Do not waste time tweaking or twiddling with sentences as it is likely that these changes will be ignored. The odd word is bound to be missing here and there – if you notice it, mark it up, but do not panic, your article will be subject to many more rounds of editorial checks. Most importantly, check that any Greek symbols are still correct (µg has a particular tendency to default to mg), decimal points are correctly placed and that any abbreviations or acronyms have been expanded accurately (particularly those relating to drug regimens). Also check the layout of all tables thoroughly. If you have been sent rough artwork to check, examine it for anatomical and labelling accuracy.

Your amended version may now be sent to the pharmaceutical company for comments; it is also likely that another editor will review it. As a result, you may be sent a further edited version and/or a further set of queries (this is why it is so important to find out who looks at what, and when, before committing yourself). When everyone is happy with the manuscript, a set of page proofs will be produced. This process is fraught with editorial dangers and you should check page proofs thoroughly (Table 15). If the errors on the proofs are a cause for concern, ask your editor to send you a revised set of pages to check. Often, the first page proofs will be the last opportunity you get to check your work. Mark any

---

Table 15
Checking page proofs

Check that:
- The text is complete and in the correct order
- Greek and mathematical symbols are correct
- Drug regimens are correct
- Figures are correctly placed (are slides/photographs correctly oriented?) and labels are accurately positioned

Unless you spot an inaccuracy:
- Do not change the text or figures
- Do not add extra text or figures

Make sure you:
- Mark your comments clearly
- Indicate amendments in the margin
- Make a copy of the pages for your files

---

amendments very, very clearly and always keep a copy. Then sit back and wait to receive a copy of the glossy final product and, of course, your cheque!

Working with a publishing company

There are two routes into the world of publishing. You may be commissioned to write a book or chapter, or you may have an idea for a medical book that you would like to pursue. Again, if approached by a commissioning editor, you should find out exactly what is involved and what your royalty will be before committing yourself. Generally, writing a book will not generate a huge income. Most authors approach publishing as a means of disseminating their expertise to a wider audience and, of course, raising their profile and establishing a reputation; the royalty cheque is a welcome bonus.

Be aware that many medical publishers sell bulk quantities of their titles to pharmaceutical companies. Although this will obviously have a considerable effect on your royalty payment, realize that, in return, the pharmaceutical company may have their name printed on the cover of the book. They will also be given the opportunity to review the manuscript and/or page proofs, and may comment accordingly. Check with your editor how much weight should be given to these comments. You will normally be free to take them on board or ignore them as you see fit; if this is not the case, you may not want to be involved with the project. For most publishers, producing a quality publication that will be valued by the reader is their priority.

If you agree to write the book, you will be sent a contract. Read it thoroughly – if any clauses cause concern, discuss them with your commissioning editor. Another good idea is to have a word with other authors who have worked with the publishing company in question; if you do not know of anyone yourself, ask the company for a few names.

If you have a startlingly original idea for a book, send an outline and details of the proposed audience to commissioning editors of various medical publishing houses. And then wait! It has to be said that few medical books start life in this way, but you could strike lucky.

Publishing is a time-consuming business. Try to get an idea of the approximate schedule from the commissioning editor at the outset, but always be prepared for delays, particularly when several authors are involved. Keep the project moving yourself, and try to meet the deadlines by writing during your 'focus time' and breaking the project up into smaller chunks.

Editing

If you are the editor or joint editor on a project, then your role may involve:

- suggesting authors for chapters
- approaching authors for contributions (or at least agreeing that letters be sent out in your name)
- suggesting a structure/chapter running order for the book or journal
- reviewing submitted chapters for suitability in terms of content and medical accuracy
- reviewing the whole publication for medical accuracy and clarity.

Although it may be tempting to do so, do not waste time laboriously correcting non-medical spelling mistakes and poor grammar. Your publisher's editor will do this. Concentrate on 'the big picture' and ask yourself whether the message is conveyed clearly and concisely to the audience you have in mind.

Further reading and resources

Albert T. Medical Journalism: *The Writer's Guide*. Oxford: Radcliffe Medical Press, 1992.

Albert T. *Winning the Publications Game: How to get Published without Neglecting your Patients*. Oxford: Radcliffe Medical Press, 1996.

Barker A. *Improve Your Communication Skills*. London: Kogan Page, 2000.

Benson J, Britten N. How much truth and to whom? Respecting the autonomy of cancer patients when talking to their families – ethical theory and the patients' view. *BMJ* 1996;313:729–31.

Buckman R. *How to Break Bad News: A Guide of Health Care Professionals*. Baltimore: Johns Hopkins University Press, 1992.

Buckman R, Kason Y. *How to Break Bad News – A Practical Guide for Healthcare Professionals*. London: Macmillan, 1993.

Conradi M, Hall R. *That Presentation Sensation*. London: Pearson Education, 2001.

Dawes K. Ghost writers need to be more visible. *BMJ* 2007;334:208.

Department of Health. *When a patient dies: Advice on developing bereavement services in the NHS.* London: DH, 2005.
http://www.dh.gov.uk/assetRoot/04/12/21/93/04122193.pdf

Fallowfield I. Giving sad and bad news. *Lancet* 1993;341:476–8.

Faulkner A. *When the News is Bad. A Guide for Health Professionals.* Nelson Thornes, 1998.

Goodman NW, Edwards MB. *Medical Writing: A Prescription for Clarity.* Cambridge: Cambridge University Press, 1991.

Gunning R. *The Technique of Clear Writing.* Revised edn. New York: McGraw Hill, 1971.

Kieffer GD. *The Strategy of Meetings.* London: Judy Piatkus, 1988.

Kirby RS. How to write a book. *Hosp Med* 2001:10 January.

Maquire P. Can communication skills be taught? *Br J Hosp Med* 1990;43:215–16.

Medicines and Healthcare products Regulatory Agency. *The Blue Guide: Advertising and Promotion of Medicines in the UK.* London: MHRA, 2005. Available to download from http://www.mhra.gov.uk/.

Meredith C, Symonds P, Webster L et al. Information needs of cancer patients in the west of Scotland. *BMJ* 1996;313:724–6.

Middleton J. *High-Impact CVs.* Oxford: Infinite Ideas, 2005.

Northouse P, Northouse LLO. Communication and cancer: issues confronting patients, health professionals and family members. *J Psychosoc Oncol* 1987;5:17–45.

Novack DH, Plumer R, Smith RI et al. Changes in physicians' attitudes toward telling the cancer patient. *JAMA* 1979;241:879–900.

O'Connor M. *Writing Successfully in Science.* London: HarperCollins, 1991.

O'Donnell M. Write for Money. In: *How to Do It.* Vol 2. London: BMJ, 1997.

Oken D. What to tell cancer patients. *JAMA* 1961;175:1120–8.

Richardson P. *A guide to medical publishing and writing.* Hospital Medicine Monograph. London: Mark Allen Publishing, 2002.

Silverman J, Kurtz S, Draper J. *Skills for Communicating with Patients.* Oxford: Radcliffe Medical Press, 1999.

Smith AJ, Preston D. Communications between professional groups in an NHS Trust hospital. *J Manage Med* 1996;10:31–9.

crisis management

'Smooth seas do not make skilled sailors'
African proverb

Although crises in medicine are much more common than in the airline business, airline personnel receive far more training in crisis management than doctors do. Knowing how to avoid, cope with and learn from crises is now an essential skill for a successful doctor. Litigation and other forms of conflict are becoming increasingly common in the NHS, and indeed throughout the world, and are more widely publicized. One major reason for this is undoubtedly poor-quality interpersonal working relationships. Part of the problem is that medical schools do not always teach students how to put medicine safely into practice and learn when mistakes are made.

Besides clinical ability, there are a number of key components of good clinical practice.

- You should practise sound clinical management. This is not only clinical ability, but means sticking to your own area of expertise and avoiding the temptation to cut corners.
- Competent and accurate administration, with scrupulous cross-checking, is integral to good clinical practice.
- Be proactive; chase the results of investigations and defaulters to make sure that those with abnormal results are followed up.
- Clear communication is essential, including the keeping of honest, accurate, up-to-date records.
- Apart from being clinically competent, a good doctor must be able to break bad news, provide counselling, obtain consent from patients for any form of intervention and generally deal kindly, honestly, professionally and effectively with people.

The difference between a consultant and a trainee is that the ultimate responsibility stops with the consultant in all of these regards. Good clinical practice and effective communication and interpersonal skills will avert most potential crises.

Complaints from patients or relatives

When something goes wrong and patients complain, it is very often because one or more of the following three key points have not been dealt with effectively:

- counselling
- consent
- breaking bad news.

It is usually problems at these levels that escalate towards litigation. When someone complains, they usually want:

- an explanation
- an apology
- rectification
- the knowledge that subsequent patients will not suffer the problem that they have experienced.

An explanation and an apology do not necessarily mean admission of guilt. The most important point here is to put a human face on the problem and to see it from the other person's point of view. The reasons may be clear to you, and it may not have been anybody's fault, but nonetheless an unfortunate outcome deserves an explanation and an apology, if only on compassionate grounds. Often a problem can be mitigated by reassuring the patient that the same thing won't happen again to somebody else. It is only occasionally that patients demand financial recompense or blood. In short, do not assume that a patient complains because they are planning to sue you for everything you've got; often the complainant simply wants to know why something happened, to hear that you regret the outcome even if it was unavoidable at the time, and to be reassured that steps will be taken to ensure that it doesn't happen again. If necessary, advice from a medicolegal specialist should be sought (see pages 159–176).

> an **unfortunate outcome** deserves an **explanation** and an **apology**

Obviously, if at all possible you should address issues and problems before they can become crises, while there is more time for information to be gathered, to prepare an appropriate response and to communicate that response effectively. There are certain characteristics that typify medical crises:

- someone is to blame, either through error or through malice, for the situation
- there is something very important at stake
- an adverse situation is brought into the open.

Clearly, certain aspects of medicine, such as working in an intensive care unit, have potential crises as part of everyday practice. However, crises that are possibly reproachable with legal action are likely to be those in which something has gone seriously wrong. Whatever the cause, a crisis is an atypical occurrence that demands an immediate response, often in the face of insufficient information and evidence. Learn to recognize the traits and weaknesses that can lead to mistakes (Table 16). In such situations, interpersonal skills are tested acutely.

Table 16
Causes of medical mistakes

Organizational
- Weak leadership
- Education/audit/research undervalued
- Cliques and factions present
- Lack of coherent strategy
- Poor communication
- Inadequate infrastructure
- Poor induction/training
- Lack of a safety culture

Personal
- Defensive attitude in the face of criticism
- Inability to learn from mistakes
- Fortress mentality
- Poor collaboration/communication
- Lack of skills
- Bad teamwork/leadership
- Poor motivation and attitude

Unfortunately, litigation is now much more common than ever before. As the level of dissatisfaction rises among hospital employees, it is inevitable that patients will be influenced by the subsequent atmosphere. Media coverage of medical 'disasters' serves only to compound this problem. Patients now have higher expectations than ever, and are not afraid to complain if these are not met.

Dealing with crises

The most important rule is to put a human face on the problem. The situation demands sympathy, understanding and, when a mistake has been made, an apology. Importantly, an expression of regret ('I'm terribly sorry this has happened') is not an admission of guilt. It is equally important to deal with the individual's perceptions ('I can see how this must seem to you') and not just the facts. Finally, as a doctor, you should remain polite, honest, caring, professional and in control at all times. Responding aggressively and defensively ('It's not my fault') is a very destructive way of dealing with such a situation. It is also vital for the whole team to learn from the mistake (see page 105 and pages 113–4).

Coping with violence

Most day-to-day violence encountered in medicine is verbal or threatened rather than physical. A dissatisfied patient may occasionally be verbally abusive, and it is important to have assistance to prevent the situation escalating. The presence of a third independent person, if only to corroborate your version of events at a subsequent enquiry, is important. If you are unsure how to respond to a verbally abusive patient, relative or member of staff, it is best to say nothing as any response might fuel their anger. Faced with silence, most people eventually run out of steam and begin to feel foolish.

Never touch an abusive person, as any form of body contact may be construed as assault, however well-meant.

Nevertheless, your duty does not extend to having to tolerate abuse of any kind. If an attempt at reasonable discussion fails, then quietly, politely, but firmly terminate the interview as soon as possible, document the occurrence carefully and inform the risk manager for the hospital trust of the events, ideally with corroboration from an independent witness. If the person concerned is a patient, notify their GP of events and suggest that the patient be referred elsewhere.

Serious physical violence in hospitals is comparatively rare, at least in Western Europe. Threatened physical violence by angry patients or by patients who are under the influence of drugs or alcohol is much more common. Broadly speaking, there are two situations. The first is when the patient is in need of urgent medical attention, in which case care should be given despite the patient's behaviour, assuming of course that it is possible to administer treatment. In the other scenario, the patient is physically threatening and not in

> your **duty** does **not** extend to **tolerating abuse**

urgent need of medical care or indeed of any treatment at all. Sometimes you may feel that enduring verbal abuse and physically threatening behaviour is part of your duty as a doctor, but you are under no obligation to do so and, if necessary, the patient can be physically removed from the hospital. However, you are obliged to point out any medical problem to the patient or to their family doctor to ensure that it is dealt with in due course.

If the patient is threatening, but not under the influence of drugs or alcohol, generally it is best to do nothing. If you remain seated and quiet, saying and doing nothing, sooner or later most patients will calm down. Never become physically threatening yourself – this only makes the situation worse. If the patient needs to be restrained, always involve hospital security staff or the police who are trained in the proper techniques – your job is to treat the patient. All hospitals now have 'risk managers' and security staff to deal with such situations.

Difficult colleagues

You can choose your friends, but you cannot choose your blood relatives or colleagues. Some so-called 'difficult colleagues' are simply people you would not choose to associate with socially. They may have their own circle of professional friends who would view you similarly. On the other hand, many hospitals have a 'difficult' employee who seems to be a law unto him- or herself. Such people usually continue to act in this way because no one has ever discussed with them the fact that their behaviour might be considered inappropriate – assuming that they are indeed a cause for concern beyond being mildly eccentric. Reasons for talking to a colleague about conduct include:

- excess alcohol consumption
- drug abuse
- actions that affect the health and safety of others, especially patients
- behaviour that may be offensive or embarrassing to others.

Some people are unaware of the effect their behaviour has on others. When an individual is confronted with this issue, he or she may respond with a torrent of abuse or aggression. Nevertheless, the best course of action is to confront the individual, bring your concerns to his or her attention and then try to address the issues. Attempting to resolve such a situation with a sympathetic discussion is greatly preferable to allowing it to escalate. It is again a question of being assertive rather than aggressive. Although such a discussion potentially may be unpleasant, if conducted politely and in an even-handed manner it is often productive.

If a colleague's behaviour continues to be a problem, particularly if substance abuse or anything that may harm patients is a factor, then you should inform the appropriate person, such as a clinical director or medical director of the trust. As a last resort you could refer the individual to the GMC (see guidance on referral of a doctor on the GMC website, http://www.gmc-uk.org/concerns/making_a_complaint/a_guide_for_health_professionals.asp#5). Your comments about colleagues must be honest and unbiased. It is better to act and then stand by a colleague as a friend than to feel that the best way of supporting them is not to report the issue. The safety of patients must be your priority at all times. Remember that your primary

the **safety** of patients must be **your priority**

duty is to your patients and other colleagues for any professional breach of conduct at work. Problems may also arise as a result of your working environment. If you have a good reason to think that patient safety may be seriously compromised by inadequate premises, equipment, or other resources, policies or systems, you should put the matter right if that is possible. In all other cases you should draw the matter to the attention of the employing or contracting body. If they do not take adequate action, you should take independent advice on how to take the matter further. You must record your concerns and the steps you have taken to try to resolve them.

Sexual harrassment

One person may feel that certain behaviour constitutes sexual harassment while another individual may consider the same a piece of harmless fun. In any relationship with patients or colleagues, you should attempt to see how your words and actions might be perceived. While most doctors are careful to consider this in their interactions with patients, they are often less observant in their relationships with colleagues. Some comments intended as 'a bit of a laugh' may not be interpreted as such by the recipient. If an individual fails to notice how badly their actions or words are received, further actions or words simply make matters worse.

Many victims of sexual (or for that matter racial) harassment tolerate it. Indeed, they may even find it amusing in small doses, and laugh about it with their colleagues; however, it is never a good idea to tolerate such behaviour, because sooner or later someone will be upset or offended. It is better to confront the individual concerned or alternatively report the matter to a third party who can take independent action. Such action might be simply to draw the matter to the attention of the wrongdoer who may desist thereafter. Indeed, some people are horrified to find that they are perceived in this way when they genuinely felt they were being friendly and amusing. More serious cases should be dealt with by a clinical or medical director. Such people should be reminded that it is not what they mean by what they say or do but how others perceive it that is important.

If you are accused of sexual harassment, what should you do? Accusations often arise from one of two situations. A patient may accuse you of harassment because they feel that you behaved inappropriately during a history taking or physical examination. For example, vaginal examination or examination of the breasts may seem inappropriate to a patient who has come to see you with backache. If you can justify your behaviour, have kept careful notes and were simply being thorough then there is unlikely to be a problem. It is possible that the patient was seen by a senior house officer or registrar, but if your name, as consultant, was on the door you will need to discuss it with the individual in person. The alternative situation is that a patient may interpret your behaviour as inappropriate based on their own perception of events, in which case it is important to view the incident from the other person's perspective. If you are accused of sexual harassment, your immediate reaction may be to attempt to justify your actions or otherwise talk your way out of the situation. The correct approach is to apologize profusely to the person your behaviour has offended and to undertake not to behave in such a way again.

If you are accused of more serious acts of sexual harassment that may contravene the standards of good behaviour set by the GMC, it is often best to say nothing until you have spoken with the medical or clinical director, your defence union or, in some cases, consulted your solicitor.

Racial and sexual discrimination

As everybody knows, racial and sexual discrimination are illegal. Although the law sets the standards by which we are expected to live, we are all aware that, in practice, these are regularly breached. On the other hand, sometimes discrimination is used as an explanation for someone not achieving a particular goal, when in fact they simply weren't up to the job.

Irrespective of racial or gender issues, favouritism (sometimes unconscious) has always existed. In our dealings with others, we should try to be fair, as we would not wish to be subject to such bias ourselves. Nowadays, anybody who is involved in interview processes will be obliged to take a course in which matters of racial and sexual discrimination are addressed. Participants will be 'trained' not to discriminate against applicants on the grounds of race, sex, religion or anything else for that matter. Application forms are being designed increasingly to exclude discrimination so far as is possible.

Bullying

Unfortunately, bullying, too, is a common problem in hospitals, although the bully may not recognize it as such. The GMC has quite rightly decreed that you must treat all your colleagues fairly and with respect. You must not bully or harass them, or unfairly discriminate against them by allowing your personal views to affect adversely your professional relationship with them. You should challenge your colleagues if their behaviour does not comply with this guidance. If you are subject to bullying from a senior colleague, do not silently accept it. Instead you should speak out, usually to your clinical director. Unless you do others will face the same torment as you, and the vicious cycle of the bullied who becomes the bully will continue.

Risk management

The possibility that an adverse event has arisen because of a more fundamental underlying problem should always be considered. This is the essence of risk management. By monitoring and learning from all unusual, unintentional or adverse events and looking for patterns in their occurrence, potential crises may be averted. This is the role of the

a **safety culture** must prevail

National Patient Safety Agency (NPSA), which has instituted an NHS-wide adverse event reporting system (http://www.npsa.nhs.uk/). Only when effective risk management exists will you be able to reassure those around you that any crisis is a one-in-a-million occurrence in an otherwise excellent track record. Remember the important dictum that 'employees may come and go but a safety culture must prevail'.

Dealing with the media following a crisis

After a recent spate of highly publicized medical disasters, it is certainly appropriate to consider how you would respond in such an unusual circumstance. One incident can spark a frenzy of antagonistic media interest, destroying, literally overnight, staff commitment that has been built up over many years.

If such a situation arises, it is essential first to establish the facts surrounding the case and obtain group support. Everyone involved in the incident should meet to develop a common understanding of what exactly has taken place and how it should be handled, otherwise the press may attempt to generate fear of a witch-hunt, encouraging staff to get their individual defensive positions on record early. Elect a spokesperson, preferably someone who has had media training or experience, to deal with the press openly and honestly. Most trusts have a designated press officer for precisely this reason. Elicit their support early on. Never attempt to go it alone.

Be wary about unsolicited telephone calls from journalists. Before answering their questions, try to find out what they know, where they got their information from and what their slant is. If possible, get your secretary to find out as much as possible about the journalist before agreeing to call back out of clinic hours. If you do have to speak to journalists, always begin by giving some sound, positive information about how the organization works, thus providing evidence that the unit normally works well and effectively (see page 80). Use other authoritative sources, such as Royal Colleges and specialist associations, to corroborate your position.

There is a tendency for doctors to bury their heads when it comes to media involvement. If you do not seize the opportunity to put good, positive news about clinical practice into the public domain, the public will only ever hear the bad news and all the good work that we do will be discounted.

Reducing medical errors

Increasingly, doctors throughout the developed world are under scrutiny, and consequently feel under pressure from politicians and especially the media. It has been estimated that 1 in every 5 patients is subject to some form of error during their hospital admission, and as many as 1 in 200 actually die as a result of iatrogenic mistakes. Currently, litigation costs the NHS more than £500 million/year, and this figure continues to rise.

What can doctors do to ensure that they themselves are not the unwilling focus of some hospital or media enquiry of a medical error affecting one (or more) of their patients? The first principle is to introduce a 'no-blame' culture of 'near-miss' error reporting. This allows doctors and other healthcare workers to learn from their mistakes and also identifies high-risk situations, which can be addressed by introducing standard operating procedures (SOPS) to reduce the chances of serious medical error; this is the major remit of the NPSA.

Secondly, it is important to understand that, when things do go badly wrong, 'system errors' are more often implicated than single mistakes by an individual. A series of minor mistakes and unfortunate coincidences usually lead up to the 'fatal error' (e.g. the removal of the wrong kidney) for which the clinician is held responsible. These 'system errors' and coincidences effectively lead the unwary into the trap of making a serious, potentially fatal mistake, or series of mistakes. This is known as an error chain.

Thirdly, warning signs of impending disaster, so-called 'red flags' (e.g. ambiguities, unease, confusion and denial) need to be recognized. Once the problem is recognized and prompt, appropriate action is taken, disaster can often be averted.

Finally, communication between clinicians and other healthcare professionals needs to be improved. Ambiguous statements such as 'remove the right (correct?) kidney' need to be avoided. Many errors in medicine occur because of mistaken identities (patients with similar names or conditions) or incompletely understood telephone conversations (sometimes in the middle of the night). Properly informed patients themselves and an insistence on feedback statements can help to avoid such difficulties. Each of us needs to develop a cross-checking mentality and be meticulous in everything we write and do, and especially what we prescribe, if we wish to avoid the trauma of serious medical error and the associated negative media coverage.

The challenge for all of us is to face up to these issues and educate ourselves, our teams, and our patients and their relatives about this important area of morbidity and mortality. Other high-risk industries, such as aviation, have already taken action by introducing Crew Resource Management courses to inform staff about how errors can be avoided. Patient safety training courses for healthcare workers may provide the way ahead. Denial that there is a problem is no longer a viable option. Clinicians should now lead the way in improving patient safety by reducing the frequency and severity of significant medical errors in their own specialty, and maintaining a safety culture within their own individual team.

Further reading and resources

Association of Trust Medical Directors. *When Things Go Wrong – Practical Steps for Dealing with the Problem Doctor.* Hingsway Cheadle: British Association of Medical Managers, 1997.

Barach P, Small SD. Reporting and preventing medical mishaps: lessons from non-medical near-miss reporting systems. *BMJ* 2000;320:753–63.

Department of Health. *Supporting doctors, protecting patients. A consultation paper on preventing, recognising and dealing with poor clinical performance of doctors in the NHS in England.* London: DH, 1999.

GMC. *Referring a doctor to the GMC: a guide for individual doctors, medical directors and clinical governance.* London: GMC, 2005.
http://www.gmc-uk.org/concerns/making_a_complaint/a_guide_for_health_professionals.asp#5

Harpwood V. *Medical Negligence and Clinical Risk: Trends and Developments.* London: Monitor Press, 1998.

Kennedy inquiry. *Report of the public inquiry into children's heart surgery at the Bristol Royal Infirmary.* London: The Stationery Office, 2001.

Kohn LT, Corrigan JM, Donaldson MS, eds. *To Err is Human: Building a Safer Health System.* Washington DC: National Academy Press, 1999.

NHS Litigation Authority. *Apologies and Explanations,* Circular 02/02. 2002.
http://www.bma.org.uk

Peason JT. Understanding adverse events: human factors. In: Vincent CA, ed. *Clinical Risk Management.* London: BMJ Publications, 1995.

Simanowitz A. Accountability. In: Vincent CA, Ennis M, Audley RJ, eds. *Medical Accidents.* Oxford: Oxford University Press, 1993:209–21.

Vincent C. *Patient Safety.* Edinburgh: Churchill Livingstone, 2006.

clinical governance and self-regulation

'Every patient who is treated in the NHS wants to know that he can rely on receiving high quality care when needed. Every part of the NHS and everyone that works in it should take responsibility for working to improve quality.'
The New NHS. Modern. Dependable, Department of Health (1997)

Clinical governance is all about quality. Until recently, quality in hospital medicine was largely related to professional self-regulation; doctors did their best and quality was the result. Now, however, this has changed. Public expectation is higher than ever before. The general level of dissatisfaction with the NHS is rising, and, as already mentioned, there have been highly publicized incidents (Bristol, Kent, Alder Hey) that have shaken public faith in the profession further. Consequently, the government is no longer happy to rely on professional self-regulation to ensure that quality standards are maintained. In fact, 'quality' itself has become an issue in recent years. In an attempt to improve the overall quality of the experience of patients undergoing medical care, the previous Conservative government introduced 'charter standards' without directly addressing the clinical issues. Various other initiatives to improve quality in clinical practice have been undertaken, such as the Confidential Enquiry into Perioperative Death, an initiative started by the Royal College of Surgeons some years ago. Indeed, the whole issue of audit was introduced to improve outcomes, and clinical outcomes in particular.

Quality has always been a major issue. So what has changed? The New Labour government introduced its plans for the health service in a document entitled *The New NHS. Modern. Dependable.* Quality issues were the central theme of the subsequent document, *A First Class Service: Quality in the New NHS.* In the original government timetable, clinical governance was to be established in 1999; the trusts reported back in

2000, showing how this has been achieved. At the same time, the National Institute for Clinical Excellence, now the National Institute for Health and Clinical Excellence (NICE) and the Commission for Health Improvement (CHI) were established and the idea of National Service Frameworks was promulgated.

The aim was to establish a national standard for quality for all the major (and many minor but expensive) clinical conditions, hence the National Service Frameworks. NICE was responsible for ensuring that national standards are set, while CHI monitored the standards by regular visits. Within each hospital trust, it became the chief executive's responsibility to ensure that clinical governance was in place to achieve the standards set nationally and monitored regionally. In each trust, a 'clinical governance group' was created to be responsible for ensuring that each directorate was doing what it should. The intention was for the entire process to be multidisciplinary, involving 'clinical teams'. Furthermore, patients' views were also to be taken into account. The National Framework for Assessing Performance would evaluate clinical performance from the patient's perspective and the Annual National Survey of Patients and User Experience would determine whether clinical services met the patients' needs. The work and bureaucracy involved in all of this was staggering.

All of this is now history. NICE still exists and functions in more or less its originally conceived form, but CHI has been replaced by CHAI and the Healthcare Commission and new agencies have sprouted, notably the National Patient Safety Agency (NPSA) with responsibilities for specific aspects of quality and safety of care.

Defining clinical governance

What does clinical governance actually mean? *A First Class Service* defines clinical governance as 'a framework through which NHS organizations are accountable for continuously improving the quality of their services and safeguarding high standards of care by creating an environment in which excellence in clinical care will flourish'. This carries both clinical and organizational obligations. Indeed, the cynic might feel that the real motive behind clinical governance is to ensure that doctors meet organizational obligations to the trust that employs them (and subsequently to the government), as well as their traditional professional and statutory obligations to their colleges and specialist associations.

The pillars of clinical governance

Some aspects of clinical governance have been components of routine clinical care for many years: audit, in particular, is established and relevant; risk management is important, albeit less familiar to doctors (but very familiar to nurses); and staff development is another well-established feature. These have been expanded into five 'pillars' of clinical governance:

- clinical audit
- clinical effectiveness
- clinical risk management
- quality assurance
- continuing staff development.

The principal difference in the way that these aspects are being approached in clinical governance currently is that the 'team' is now the focus rather than the doctor; and the entire 'clinical experience' is being monitored rather than patients' treatment by the doctor specifically. Therefore, all points of contact between the hospital and the patient – sometimes referred to as 'the patient journey' – are addressed. It includes outpatients in the accident and emergency department, the ambulance service, the admission process, the ward as a physical environment, the domestic services, the nursing care, the care provided by other healthcare professionals and the medical care; every aspect is taken into account. The 'team' includes doctors, nurses, physiotherapists, dietitians, pharmacists, secretaries and anyone responsible for a particular 'clinical experience' or 'patient journey'.

Clinical audit

Doctors have been involved in clinical audit for sometime, although many specialties have never taken it very seriously. In clinical audit, performance within a given area is monitored and compared with others' performances; reasons that account for any difference are then identified. A mechanism can then be put in place to improve performance, and reassessment should confirm that a better outcome has been achieved. It is this latter component of audit – 'closing the loop', as it is called – that doctors have often been rather lax at addressing. Audit in hospitals has so far been entirely clinical. Doctors have worked out the best ways to approach and report the audit they wanted to undertake. Now, hospital managers want to be assured that audit topics are comprehensive, the activities selected for audit in each directorate are systematic and findings are acted upon. Audit must address all the important quality issues with the goal of improved overall quality of care and particular reference to patient experience and outcome. In other words, it must be open and accountable to outsiders.

clinical audit must address all the important quality issues

Clinical effectiveness

Clinical effectiveness may be best defined colloquially as 'doing the right thing right'. Recent interest in effectiveness has centred on evidence-based clinical practice. A number of books and databases – particularly the Cochrane databases – have developed around the theme of evidence-based medicine. Clearly, the idea is very sound. There is no point in providing a treatment, particularly an invasive procedure, if it is ineffective, however well it is administered. Evaluating clinical effectiveness will ensure that ineffective treatments are identified and discontinued, and effective treatments are administered to the highest possible standard. One way of achieving this is to make sure that patients follow so-called 'care pathways', and that outcomes are monitored against the accepted national standards referred to previously.

Some critics argue that much of the evidence obtained in this way is not 'medicine-based evidence'. Although evidence-based medicine is all very well for clear-cut medical problems in uncomplicated cases, this is often not the case in real life. Indeed, many patients are excluded from the clinical trials on which evidence-based medicine is based for precisely this reason. 'Case mix' is therefore an important factor in the interpretation of clinical effectiveness, particularly when an external authority may judge consultants on the outcome of their activities. It is argued that doctors will not want to treat complicated patients if they are to be judged by the same standards as those doctors who treat the straightforward cases. In practice, evaluating clinical effectiveness is not a case of simply monitoring morbidity and mortality, but of finding out whether treatments were appropriate and effective for a patient's specific clinical circumstances. There are many examples of treatment, in both medicine and surgery, that may occasion neither morbidity nor mortality but which make no difference to the course or outcome of a clinical condition – usually at some expense.

Clinical risk management

By recognizing and reviewing the adverse events that occur, we can identify ways to prevent them. The goal of risk management is to reduce the occurrence and the consequences of adverse events. For some time, risk management in hospitals has been associated with health and safety. Anything that is not a part of routine patient care or organizational activity is documented as an 'incident', and these incidents are analysed on a regular basis. The analysis serves to identify any underlying patterns that may suggest a more fundamental problem that needs to be addressed. A national reporting system has been proposed by the NPSA (http://www.npsa.nhs.uk/). Most incidents are relatively trivial until an incident presents in a slightly different form so as to be termed a crisis. Incidents (within the definition given) can be identified by anybody working within an organization. On the whole, they tend to be reported by nurses, who are in closer contact with patients

> evaluating **clinical effectiveness** is **not** simply monitoring **morbidity** and **mortality**

and are much more familiar with the concepts of risk management and health and safety.

Other points for consideration in risk management include specific points raised by patients, usually in letters of complaint. These need to be read not just for the particular complaint but also as a means of identifying underlying problems that may be of a more serious nature. Any defects or drawbacks identified should be actively corrected and cross-checked to ensure patient safety has been established and is maintained.

The aim of clinical risk management is to apply these ideas more specifically to patient care. All members of the clinical team must be encouraged to identify and report adverse events – so-called 'free lessons' (see the Heinrich Ratio, Figure 6) – enabling everyone to learn from such experiences in a blame-free way. The ultimate goal is a reduced risk of adverse events, and therefore improved patient care. The most obvious clinical improvement would be a reduction in the incidence of iatrogenic disease, including pharmacological errors, which has been estimated to cost the NHS more than £2 billion each year (Table 17).

identify and report
free lessons

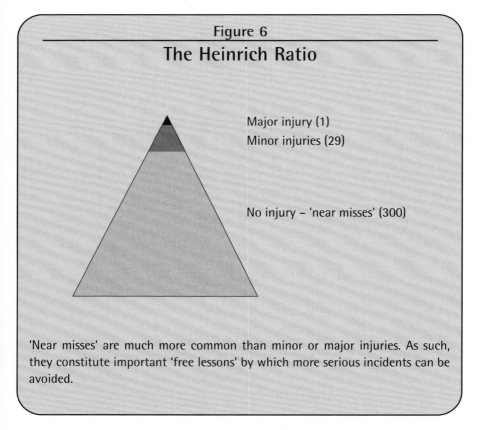

Figure 6
The Heinrich Ratio

Major injury (1)
Minor injuries (29)

No injury – 'near misses' (300)

'Near misses' are much more common than minor or major injuries. As such, they constitute important 'free lessons' by which more serious incidents can be avoided.

Table 17

Estimated annual cost of iatrogenic disease to the NHS

- £2 billion due to lost bed days
- £500 million resulting from medical negligence claims
- 6600 serious device-related incidents reported
- 9800 serious drug reactions reported

Quality assurance

There is a considerable overlap between quality assurance and clinical effectiveness, and of course both are intimately involved in clinical audit. Quality assurance is principally concerned with the monitoring and measurement of performance against standards, rather than the less rigorous assessments of clinical audit. Quality assurance programmes are particularly important in screening programmes, pathology, blood transfusion and radiology. In clinical practice, good examples of quality assurance include proper practice in keeping patient records, prescribing and administering treatments appropriately, and completing diagnostic coding.

Quality assurance is not, however, a static process. Over the last few years, the Modernisation Agency has sought to drive initiatives to improve the patient journey and otherwise look at new and potentially better or more cost-effective ways of delivering care and providing a service. The Modernisation Agency has now been disbanded as a central organization within the Department of Health and its staff and activities have been devolved downwards so that service development is now an integral component of all NHS Trusts.

Staff development

In many professions, staff development or continuing professional development, including a regular appraisal process, is standard and well established. Regular appraisals are now widely regarded as an integral part of getting the best out of the personnel of any business. In contrast, until recently, staff development in the health service has largely been a passive process. Doctors were appointed to a post, stayed in it until the end of that particular appointment and then moved on. Unless they were particularly good or particularly bad, nobody took much notice of their performance during that time. However, appraisals and assessments for trainees have been introduced, and now consultants must provide evidence of continuing medical education to demonstrate that they are keeping abreast of recent developments. Poor performance has been brought to the forefront in cases such as that involving paediatric cardiac surgery in Bristol (Table 18), illustrating that an adequate knowledge base on its own, which is probably the best that continuing medical education alone can provide, is insufficient. The consultant must have adequate clinical and non-clinical skills on which to draw if he or she is to provide a sufficiently good overall performance. In the case of a surgeon or interventionist, this includes both technical operative skills and intraoperative decision-making. Although all doctors have their own particular clinical skills, they also have non-clinical skills that are common to all specialties. In particular, these concern counselling, breaking bad news, communicating with patients and staff, dealing with problems and relating well to other people. These interpersonal skills are probably more important to an average patient than the clinical skills. Likewise, poor clinical performance is not just carrying out an operation badly or giving the wrong drug dose or treatment, but also poor record-keeping, poor communication, disruptive working behaviour or simply the inability to work as part of a team.

The 'job plan' is a tool used to identify what a consultant actually does. Completed annually, it has simply documents the average working week of a consultant – ward rounds, outpatient clinics, operating lists and other 'professional activities' (PAs) plus on-call duties, administration, research, audit, examining, teaching and committee attendance. These are divided into PAs for direct clinical care and PAs for supporting activities, with the obvious expectation that although the specific nature of PAs for direct clinical care may vary from consultant to consultant they will nonetheless form the bulk of the job plan, with PAs for supporting activities forming the rest. The job plan is completed by the consultant and signed off in turn by the clinical director and by the medical director, and forms part of the overall process of annual appraisal of each consultant by his or her

Clinical governance and self-regulation

Table 18

The Bristol cardiac surgery case

The Bristol case involved a team of cardiac surgeons working in Bristol and concerned their performance of a particular type of 'switch' surgery used for the treatment of a specific congenital malformation. This operation was established as the standard of care, but in order to achieve consistently good results, a very high standard of surgical technique is required, together with scrupulous preoperative evaluation and postoperative care. A national register of these operations had been established sometime before and so the overall mortality was known as a baseline against which individual results could be judged.

It had become apparent that the results in Bristol were substantially worse (mortality was double that of other units) than the national register suggested they should be, and it also became apparent that the parents of the children involved had been given unrealistic expectations of what surgery could achieve. Furthermore, although the results at Bristol had been pointed out to various authorities and to the surgeons themselves, the surgeons had continued to operate and no effective action had been taken to deal with the issues that had arisen.

This raised a number of questions in relation to clinical standards, audit and the comparison of individual surgeons' results against a generally accepted national standard: how and by whom individual doctors' performance is monitored; the responsibility of individual consultants in relation to their own performance; the honesty with which risks are explained to patients; the need to protect patients from doctors who are 'in difficulty' (in any sense of the phrase); and, most difficult, how to assess technical expertise and clinical competence, particularly in advanced procedures. The last has obvious implications for training: how can doctors work competently while on the inevitable 'learning curve' when undertaking new procedures, and how should doctors be trained to perform difficult advanced procedures which are not part of routine practice? The Royal Colleges, specialist associations and individual NHS Trusts are currently trying to address these issues.

clinical director or other nominated individual. The job plan, clinical activity, professional and patient-related interpersonal relationships, continuing professional development, health, probity and other governance-related activities (audit and clinical effectiveness) all form part of this process. This may be viewed as a procedure aimed primarily at identifying and reporting poor performance. Although this is undoubtedly one reason for the exercise, there is nonetheless a positive side to clinical professional development in the widest sense. It must be remembered that identifying poor performance is a valuable goal in itself, particularly if it prevents harm. Regular annual appraisal will be an important component of revalidation, as discussed below.

Revalidation of doctors' registration

As a result of adverse publicity, the GMC decided that doctors must demonstrate, on a regular basis, that they are up-to-date and fit to practise in their chosen field. Doctors who fail to show this competence will lose their registration.

The revalidation of registration is the biggest single change to medical regulation since the Medical Act set up the GMC in 1958. As a result, the medical register has become a record of a doctor's continuing fitness to practise rather than a historical record of qualifications acquired in training. Although doctors' revalidation will be recorded centrally and publicly through the GMC's registers, quality assurance of an individual's performance will be monitored at a local level.

The precise details of how to deliver revalidation are still the subject of detailed discussion, although it is clear that regular satisfactory annual appraisal is central to the whole process. Indeed, at the time of publication the planned introduction of revalidation has been deferred pending yet another report and consultation. In July 2006, the Department of Health published *Good doctors, safer patients: Proposals to strengthen the system to assure and improve the performance of doctors and to protect the safety of patients. A report by the Chief Medical Officer.* One major bone of contention is the recommendation to change the standard of proof from the criminal standard to the civil standard, effectively lowering the threshold of proof required before a finding can be made on the facts of a case. This would have the effect of making it easier for the GMC to prove allegations against doctors and result in more erasures from the medical register, which is to be deplored. There are many other sensitive issues, in particular whether it is right for NHS management to become deeply involved in assessing the clinical skills and knowledge of doctors. The combination of revalidation and managerial quality assurance, such as clinical governance, promises to reassure the public that robust systems are in place to monitor and support doctors in their work. These systems also serve to demonstrate that the majority of doctors, who are both able and conscientious, reach the high standards required of them.

Your part in clinical governance

At this stage, the most important thing to do is get involved with the clinical governance programme being developed by your trust and your directorate. Work together with all your colleagues, looking at what you do together, how you do it and how well you do it.

Deaths and complications meetings are a good channel for focussing on clinical problems, but remember to focus on the wider aspects of these problems. Take particular note of nursing and other paramedical activities, adverse incidents and patient complaints. Find out what you can do to reduce the risk of all adverse events.

Evidence-based best practice should be identified. Audit your own activities to make sure best practice is followed and national standards of performance achieved. Aim to identify and discontinue ineffective treatments or other wasteful practices. When problems of an

> find out what you can do to reduce the risk of adverse events

organizational or managerial nature arise, make hospital management aware. This includes faulty equipment, insufficient staffing, poor hospital fabric and any other organizational aspect that adversely affects clinical practice.

Within the framework of clinical governance itself, the single biggest barrier is adequate information. This is closely followed by increasingly insufficient time to process and analyse this information. It is certainly true that for sophisticated analysis and results that will stand up to rigorous external scrutiny, information technology in most trusts is currently woefully inadequate. Nonetheless, most of the general points outlined here can be addressed without recourse to sophisticated information technology, and you are likely to benefit if the principles of clinical governance are approached with an open mind.

Most importantly, remember that you are not working in splendid isolation but as part of a team, and that people around you will begin to take more of an interest in what you do than they ever have done before. Clinical governance is a train coming down the track. You could try to stop it by standing in the way, or you could move aside, but be left behind. The best policy is to leap aboard and make it one of the vehicles of your own as well as your institution's success.

Further reading and resources

Burke C, Lugon M. *Integrating clinical risk and clinical audit – moving towards clinical governance.* Healthcare Risk Resource 1998;2:16–18.

Department of Health. *The New NHS. Modern. Dependable.* Cm 3807. London: DH, 1997.
http://www.archive.official-documents.co.uk/document/doh/newnhs/contents.htm

Department of Health. *A First Class Service: Quality in the New NHS.* London: DH, 1998.
http://www.dh.gov.uk/PublicationsAndStatistics/Publications/PublicationsPolicyAnd
Guidance/PublicationsPolicyAndGuidanceArticle/fs/en?CONTENT_ID=4006902&chk=j2
Tt7C

Department of Health. *Good doctors, safer patients: Proposals to strengthen the system to assure and improve the performance of doctors and to protect the safety of patients. A report by the Chief Medical Officer.* 276071. London: DH, 2006.
http://www.dh.gov.uk/assetRoot/04/13/72/76/04137276.pdf

General Medical Council. *Revalidating Doctors: Ensuring Standards, Securing the Future.* London: GMC, 2000.

Halligan A, Donaldson L. Implementing clinical governance: turning vision into reality. *BMJ* 2001;322:1413–17.

Irvine D. The performance of doctors. 1. Professionalism and self-regulation in a changing world. *BMJ* 1997;314:1540–2.

Kennedy inquiry. *Report of the public inquiry into children's heart surgery at the Bristol Royal Infirmary.* London: The Stationery Office, 2001.

Lugon M, Secker-Walker J. *Clinical Governance: Making it Happen.* London: Royal Society of Medicine Press, 1999.

Lugon M, Secker-Walker J, eds. *Advancing Clinical Governance*. London: Royal Society of Medicine Press, 2001.

Miles A, Hampton J, Hurwitz B, eds. *NICE, CHI and the NHS Reforms: Enabling Excellence or Imposing Control?* London: Key Advances, 2000.

Report of an Expert Group on Learning from Adverse Events in the NHS. *An Organisation with a Memory*. London: The Stationery Office, 2000.

Wright J, Hill P. *Clinical Governance*. Edinburgh: Churchill Livingstone, 2003.

management

Keith Parsons FRCS
Consultant Urological Surgeon, Past Chief Executive of the
Royal Liverpool and Broadgreen University Hospitals NHS Trust

*'Take two managers and give to each the same number of
laborers and let those laborers be equal in all respects. Let both
managers rise equally early, go equally late to rest, be equally
active, sober, and industrious, and yet, in the course of the year,
one of them, without pushing the hands that are under him more
than the other, shall have performed infinitely more work.'*
George Washington (1732–1799)

In the mid-1980s the government of the day realized that the National
Health Service, which had improved healthcare provision comprehensively
in the postwar years, could potentially run out of control. Its clarity of
purpose and the dedication of its staff were not questioned, but how it delivered services and at what cost appeared an impenetrable mystery. The mismatch between demand and resources was becoming evident, and the potential to consume more and more of the gross national product seemed a real risk.

> it was once **understood** that the **NHS** was **unlikely** to **meet all demands**

As a first step to introduce some sort of order in the face of
unrestricted spending, the Chancellor introduced cash-limited budgets for
the NHS. Initially cash limits applied only to the hospital sector, but soon
they were extended to include the whole of the NHS. This rather blunt
instrument began to exert control on spending, but the problem of
reconciling services with costs remained.

In the early years of the NHS, there had been an implicit understanding that the service was unlikely to meet all demands made on it. Indeed, queues were common, waiting lists were accepted, the service was run by administrators, and politics were not involved. Intriguingly, the minister responsible did not have a place in the Cabinet. The financial imperative introduced in the 1980s meant that the previous scheme, which had served the NHS so well, was unlikely to be adequate for the new fiscal rigour. An executive from a large supermarket chain was asked to produce a report on the NHS from his background and perspective and to make suggestions for change. The interim 9-page letter that was produced became known as the Griffiths Report. A formal document was never produced but it was this little report that drew attention to the fact that the NHS was not *managed*, and that for any prospect of improvement, or indeed its very survival, it would have to be.

As might be imagined, the medical profession perceived management as a huge threat, an impingement on the right to independent practice and a generally impudent suggestion. Yet management techniques and expertise were introduced, and the report proved a turning point for the NHS. It took the better part of 10 years from those first steps for anything like a coherent management system to evolve; sceptics might hold that coherence is still awaited.

The concept that more management was good for the NHS has, to say the least, not been universally and enthusiastically embraced by the medical profession. The problem has been threefold. Firstly, there was an inherent mistrust by the medical profession of managers, whom they saw as 'outsiders' with little knowledge of medicine invading hallowed medical territory. Maybe the initial implementation the Griffiths Report was to blame. A large number of managers from industry and elsewhere were imported to run health authorities and hospitals. This was not a successful experiment, and of the 164 health authority external appointees, those still in post after 3 years could be counted on the fingers of one hand.

changes have been **imposed** roughly **every 5 years**

Secondly, the temptation to reorganize regularly was not resisted. Far from leaving the NHS to evolve and develop, substantial organizational changes have been imposed roughly every 5 years. These are usually heralded as major improvements, though the latest is accompanied by the mantra *modernization*.

Finally politicians have put the NHS firmly in the political arena, with a Secretary of State most prominent in the Cabinet and general elections allegedly won or lost on healthcare policy.

Fortunately, managerial appointments are now much more attuned to the requirements of running successful healthcare organizations. Why is this a good thing and why are managers such crucial element to modern healthcare in the NHS? The successful hospital doctor needs to know.

The business of health

Whether we like it or not, the NHS has to be a managed system. It is not a democracy and must actively avoid responding to only the strongest vested interest. In the past, the NHS has often made both mistakes. It has to meet the demands of elected government, who are in turn accountable to the electorate, and the needs of those who use the service.

Expenditure in the NHS accounts for a significant and increasing proportion of the UK's gross domestic product, currently some 7.1%. An announcement by the Chancellor in the budget in April 2002 committed the country to continuing increase in NHS funding. The plan is to double healthcare spending over the next 10 years and to better the European average. It should perhaps not go unnoticed that the driver for this policy was another externally

the **NHS** has to be **managed**

commissioned study, the Wanless Report, this one written by the retired chief executive of a high-street bank.

Spending taxpayers' money in such large amounts cannot be a random process. Knowing what is delivered and how and the ways in which this can be improved is the very essence of management. We should all contribute enthusiastically and energetically to this process if we are to retain the cooperation of our patients and see real improvements for them, and there appears now to be a continuing opportunity for this to happen.

Understanding the management structure

Successful doctors should be familiar with the management structure of the NHS Trust in which they work. This will equip them with the necessary tools to effect change and improvements in patient care when needed, and enable them to foster a spirit of collaboration and cooperation.

To get to grips with the management structure, it is important to understand the basic differences between executive and governance functions.

Executive management and governance

A board of executive and non-executive directors manages every NHS Trust, with every director of equal status. Executive directors are responsible for the day-to-day management of the trust. Non-executive directors are notable members of the local community appointed to the trust board by the Secretary of State for Health. They must ensure that the executives perform their duties within the requirements of a public body and, in so doing, they fulfil their governance function.

The entire board sets the strategy for the trust, and the chief executive must see that the strategy is enacted; the trust chairman, a non-executive director, ensures that this process takes place. The chairman is responsible directly to the Secretary of State, although regular contact with the NHS Executive is through the Regional Chairman. In April 2003, regional executive and local health authorities were replaced by Strategic Health Authorities, which are responsible for the liaison between Primary Care Trusts (PCTs) and NHS Trust hospitals and set strategies responsive to the needs of the local population and to meet Government targets, for example those required by National Service Frameworks or to comply with minimum waiting times.

> the **chief executive** sees that the **strategy** is enacted

Below board level, each NHS Trust will have a slightly different management structure, within which each service discipline has a line-management responsibility to the chief executive and the board. This management responsibility is different from the professional responsibility of doctors, which is determined by the General Medical Council.

Most service disciplines are structured as clinical directorates with a clinical director who is responsible to the chief executive. Remember that clinical directors do a lot, but what they do not do is direct clinically! Many will have had some management training, so if an opportunity to become a clinical director arises, do not hold back from accepting, but insist that appropriate management training is made available to you. The recommendations of the Redfearn Report into organ retention at Alder Hey Hospital in Liverpool make this quite clear. This report criticized firstly those doctors who were in a position with managerial responsibility who had no specific training and secondly had harsh words for those who were managing in areas outside their clinical specialty. The answer, of course, is quite simple – accept a clinical director's post only in your own discipline, and be sure to be trained at least to a basic level in management techniques before accepting responsibility.

> accept a **clinical director's post** only in **your own discipline**

Funding

The funding stream upon which any hospital relies is now controlled and managed by the PCTs. They are responsible for commissioning healthcare for the population which they serve. In the modernization agenda, a new scheme of referral to hospital is being introduced in which patients have the right to choose from a list of providers. On that list will be providers in the private sector, though any charges will be responsibility of the PCTs, thus retaining the principle that NHS healthcare remains free for the patient at the point of delivery. It remains to be seen whether this 'Choice' scheme is a success.

There is a further new feature relating to NHS Trusts in the modernization agenda; namely, some hospitals are granted a degree of financial independence in return for reaching a quality standard determined on financial results and clinical star ratings. These 'Foundation Hospitals' will thrive or otherwise depending upon their performance. The hypothesis is that the freedom from central control will encourage better performance.

Accountability

The chief executive is accountable, ultimately to Parliament, for the organization. This accountability is through the Chief Executive of the NHS, who is himself accountable through the system of Parliamentary Select Committees – either the Select Committee on Health or the Public Accounts Committee.

There are four broad areas for which the chief executive is held to account:

- achieving financial balance
- meeting a predetermined return on the capital asset of the trust
- operating within the external funding limit for the trust
- maintaining clinical standards.

The first three are purely financial responsibilities, but the fourth is managed in most trusts by the mechanism and processes of clinical governance. The performance is then reflected in a star rating system, many of the components of which depend upon clinical achievements. No stars is bad and three stars is as good as it can get.

Clinical governance

This does not involve any manager in a direct executive role in patient management, but is a requirement that ensures that all clinicians, not just doctors, deliver healthcare to the trust's patients at a level required by a public body. It is a mechanism whereby the chief executive can be reassured that the clinicians in the trust are performing optimally. It is not at all unreasonable for the accountable officer to require such reassurance. The clinical governance processes in each trust may differ slightly, but they should not be a threat but an opportunity for healthcare professions. Clinical governance should ensure that the circumstances in which clinicians work are appropriate, and this is an unquestionable

clinical governance ensures **healthcare delivery** at a **required level**

responsibility of the trust. In return, the clinical services which healthcare professionals provide must fulfil all the requirements of good practice, undoubtedly the clinicians' responsibility. This symbiotic relationship should be used in the context of continuous quality improvement and facilitate raising standards in all clinical areas. The most successful doctors will grasp its concepts eagerly.

How to manage

First, forget administration; the NHS is too complex and important to be merely administered. Administration is a completely inadequate concept for modem healthcare. It breeds bureaucracy, slowness and pedantry, and stifles imaginative and innovative thinking. A hospital is a complex organization, in which a great number of people, including those treated by it and who work for it, have a diverse range of requirements. Nowadays, most city hospitals employ the equivalent of the population of a small town and annually may see a total number of patients equivalent to the population of a provincial city. Indeed, if visitors are also taken into consideration, the number of people coming through the hospital doors each year may match the population of Denmark! Consequently, an enormous range of requirements are generated, from simple procurement functions to complex interactions of, for example, employment law, health and safety legislation, fire regulations, design technology, informatics and data protection, to name but a few. Each of these elements has no direct reference to medical interactions, yet all are vital in ensuring that patients receive the highest quality treatment. It is essential that all of these aspects are managed with authority and skill.

the **number of people** coming through the doors **each year** may match the **population of Denmark**

Not everybody is interested in management, but in the end either you become involved or you are managed by somebody else. Generally, it is better to be involved yourself.

Probably the most important management decisions concern:

- setting priorities
- planning to achieve them
- maintaining the quality of the service provided as a consequence.

view the NHS from a concerned relative's perspective

It is impossible to underestimate the importance of quality. Put yourself in the place of a worried relative or sick patient and you will quickly realize that a high-quality service is paramount, queues and delays are unacceptable, and an almost guaranteed outcome most desirable. Viewing the NHS from a concerned relative's perspective will help you appreciate the importance of these factors.

Managing change

As the consultant lead of a clinical team, the clinical director in management, or indeed in any other area such as a professional association, remember the importance of informing people how a change will be effected, what purpose the change serves, and their responsibilities during the changes. Similarly, when change has been brought about, remind others of what has been done and why. Keeping people well informed makes them more likely to comply, because they feel involved. Your colleagues will generally be grateful that somebody else is doing the managing; however, always listen and be careful not to make them feel their opinions are not wanted. Keep talking to them throughout, reminding them collectively what is being done.

Undoubtedly, the medical profession has been challenged to 'modernize'. This word is used widely in the NHS and means whatever the user, like Humpty Dumpty, wishes it to mean. Yet often imaginative and progressive-thinking doctors are held back. The innovative and successful are those who can see a vision, engineer change and stick at it, bringing their colleagues along with them.

If the attributes of a good clinical director were to be prioritized, vision, leadership and the ability to take decisions would certainly be the top three.

Effective management

As a general rule, doctors should make good managers. Our very training requires us to respond immediately to potential clinical catastrophes with authoritative management. The discipline, clarity of thought and authority of action needed to approach the day-to-day situations in which doctors find themselves are not so very different from the requirements of an effective manager.

doctors should make **good managers**

A clinical manager must recognize that what is required is relatively simple. Workload, personnel and budget, the essence of all business plans, whether for the biggest corporation or the smallest clinical directorate, have to be reconciled. The 'kiss' principle certainly applies – Keep It Simple, Stupid!

Working with your manager colleagues

It is a grave mistake to underestimate the commitment of NHS managers to the health service and the institutions in which they work. They are as important to successful patient care as any other professional group in the hospital. Generally, NHS managers have many years of experience and have worked extensively at different management levels in health authorities, hospitals and elsewhere. It is essential to remember that everyone is working towards a common goal.

The dangers of intellectual arrogance

To be considered inferior and then to demonstrate otherwise is a powerful and disarming weapon, and some managers will use this readily. Always avoid assuming intellectual superiority – it is better not to run the risk of being caught in this simple trap and made to look foolish.

avoid assuming **intellectual superiority**

Don't hide behind clinical imperative

It can be tempting to raise the clinical imperative argument to get your own way. 'My patients must have this or they will suffer appallingly' has been heard all too commonly, often unjustified by the clinical circumstance. No doubt there are times when you will make demands on behalf of your patients – do so in an intelligent and thoughtful way that engages proper discussion. If you try the old technique of shroud-waving, you will find that you get away with it only once or twice.

Money matters

You might be forgiven for thinking that money does not matter, but since the NHS became cash-limited, it is of fundamental importance. We should be as cost-efficient as possible in all that we do. Everything done for patients has a cost implication, and we must ensure that maximum benefit is achieved for as many as possible. Since politicians make the ultimate decision on total healthcare expenditure, they are responsible for rationing. It is the clinicians' responsibility to direct that expenditure; the more effectively and efficiently this is done, the better the management relationship will become.

Take an interest in where the money comes from

Never forget that it is taxpayers' money that the NHS spends. A good manager will treat the organization's money as carefully as if it were his or her own.

It is all too easy for doctors to stand back and let others struggle with the complexities of commissioning healthcare, and then criticize the outcome. PCTs are making the relationship between primary and secondary care more complicated than ever before. Some 75% of the total NHS budget will be handed to PCTs to manage, and thus they will have a profound influence on the future shape of health services.

> a **good manager** will treat the organization's **money carefully**

Words may change and sentiments alter, but there will always be a need for hospitals to determine what they can deliver and demands from primary care to deliver more at a lower cost. Successful doctors will be interested in this process and assist wherever possible. Contracts and finance departments need help, so collaborate with them when you can, especially in discussions with PCTs.

Yet another element of modernization is the 'payment by results' principle. This will require even closer cooperation between the clinical and managerial teams, so clearly those who are good at this are likely to do well and those who are not, will not. There is a pressing need to understand the new relationship between hospitals and general practitioners, who will have more influence on policy and direction in the future. When the rationing debate is considered, as inevitably it will be, this relationship will become still more relevant.

Beware the zero-sum game argument

It is easy to assume that any development in a limited resource system has to be paid for by shifting resources from elsewhere – which is true, to some extent. But Paul doesn't always have to be paid by a robbed Peter. If you are innovative in your thinking, there are often ways to fund new developments that do not require simple transfer of money from one project to another. Be imaginative and discuss the alternatives with your manager colleagues; it is likely that you will find a most receptive ear. In industry, there are no doubt thousands of examples of very simple measures that have released resources. One of the most impressive was that of a worker at the Bryant and May match company who suggested putting sandpaper on one side of the box only rather than both. This simple suggestion saved the company millions of pounds. There is no reason why similar suggestions should not apply in medicine. Those most likely to identify such initiatives are those working closest to patients.

Demand evidence-based management

Management is a sophisticated science, and those working in this field are professionals. They will respect a legitimate challenge, and you should demand the same standards from your management colleagues as you do from other medical professionals. It is not unreasonable to ask for evidence to support the management's propositions. Evidence will undoubtedly be provided, but the subsequent discussion will serve to focus both parties and ultimately enhance the outcome. A track record of working in this way will result in managers turning to you first when they need help with making difficult decisions.

Recognize corporate responsibility

There still is only one NHS, for which we all work.

Conflicts of interest

In some cases, it will be impossible to meet both the needs of an individual patient and the patient population as a whole, and you may need to make decisions about use of resources and provision of patient care. There is no simple solution when caught on the horns of this dilemma. You must consider the priorities of the government, the NHS and your trust. As a clinician, however, the care of your patient must be your first concern, bearing in mind the consequences that your decision will have on the available resources and the choices of other patients. Your responsibility as a manager and doctor is to allocate resources in a way that best serves the interests of the community or entire patient population. In both capacities, you will make the best decision by using the best evidence from research and audit.

> use the **evidence** from **research** and **audit**

Protecting patients from harm

As a doctor and manager, you must take action if you believe that patients are at serious risk of harm. The GMC now make this the duty of a doctor, and *not* to act may be construed as professional misconduct. Concerns about safety may arise from the result of critical incident reporting, clinical audit, complaints from patients or information provided by colleagues. If you receive such

> **take action** if you believe that **patients** are at **serious risk**

information, you must act on it. As a manager, it will be necessary for you to establish the facts before taking action yourself. Alternatively, you may need to report the concerns to your own manager or a senior colleague.

Dealing with colleagues

If your responsibilities include managing colleagues, ensure that procedures are in place for dealing with their concerns and that all staff are made aware of them. As a manager, you must be prepared to discuss problems that your staff encounter in their professional capacity both sympathetically and constructively. It is a requirement that an annual appraisal is undertaken of each consultant staff member so that their GMC registration can be revalidated. It is thus important that you are properly trained in appraisal technique. Appraisal should not be a mechanism of policing competence; rather, it should be used to support doctors, but you must also be willing

> **appraisal** should be used to **support doctors**

to take any necessary action should serious problems emerge. All concerns should be investigated, documented and, if found genuine, acted upon following discussions with other colleagues and senior managers. The protection of patients should remain the driving force at all times.

Pride and prejudice

Politics are a fact of life in the NHS. Difficult as it may be to accept, both doctors and managers will always be subject to the frustrations of working in a politically driven healthcare delivery system. The best mechanism for dealing with this is to work together, recognizing and striving to meet the particular demands that the system creates. The alternative is to take entrenched opposing positions, but this only wastes time and energy.

Perhaps the greatest satisfaction that successful doctors can have is recognition of their worth, so take pride in your hospital and make the board proud of you. Taking pride in the institution in which you work is a good starting point. Behind the facade of league tables and benchmarking lies the real issue of working for your local team. This has wider implications from a strategic standpoint. If you get this right, everyone associated with your institution will take pride in what you achieve.

Further reading and resources

Young AE. *The Medical Manager*, 2nd edn. Oxford: Blackwell, 2003.

finance

Andrew CD Lang FCA
Sandison Lang & Co Chartered Accountants

'Annual income twenty pounds, annual expenditure nineteen pounds, nineteen shillings and six, result happiness. Annual income twenty pounds, annual expenditure twenty pounds ought and six, result misery'
Mr Micawber in *David Copperfield*, Charles Dickens (1850)

Traditionally, doctors have not really focussed on financial matters. The assumption has always been that medicine is an intellectually and financially satisfying vocation. Many regard simply qualifying as a doctor as a guarantee of financial success; beyond that, they feel there is no need to worry about the slightly unsavoury issue of money. In fact, the reverse is true: financial security breeds success and success breeds financial security.

financial security breeds success

To begin on a good footing, always be scrupulously honest in financial and commercial matters related to your work. It is also important to avoid accumulating substantial debts. There are, however, two exceptions for which it is acceptable to take on a debt: taking on a student loan for training; and borrowing for a short overseas placement in the form of an elective while you are a student or junior doctor. A student loan enables you to qualify; once this is achieved, overseas visits can broaden your outlook, provide invaluable clinical experience and enhance your CV, giving selection committees something to discuss in your first crucial interviews. Beg or borrow – but do not steal – the money needed for either or both of these!

The early years

Following qualification, your first hospital appointment will provide a regular monthly salary; spending and saving wisely at this time will provide solid foundations for the future.

Buying property

Property has long been regarded as one of the safest investments over the years. To maximize capital appreciation, the sooner you can step onto the property ladder, the better. Consider taking the largest possible mortgage at the outset; as your income rises, the mortgage repayments will represent a lower percentage of your net income. The three main options for repaying the mortgage are outlined in Table 19.

> the **sooner** you can **step** onto the **property ladder**, the **better**

Renting property

Rental payments are often money wasted – the money could be put towards a mortgage. If your employment requires that you change location every year or so, as is often the case with junior doctors, you could rent out your property on a short-term basis to recoup the mortgage repayments. Hospital trusts will often pay your removal expenses.

Long-term sickness/critical illness insurance

Under the terms of the NHS Superannuation Scheme, in the event of sickness or illness you will receive:
- full salary for the first 6 months of incapacity
- half salary for the next 6 months.

After 1 year of permanent disability, the benefits depend on the number of years of NHS service, which are unlikely to be significant at this stage of your career. You would therefore be strongly advised to consider taking out your own sickness policy; the sooner you do this, the cheaper

Table 19

Mortgages

Repayment mortgage
- The capital and interest are paid off over an agreed period of years (usually 25 years)
- The initial payments are mostly interest on the loan, but as the sum borrowed declines, a greater fraction of the regular payment goes towards repaying the capital
- Repayment mortgages are available in various forms to suit different financial situations: some have a fixed interest rate for the first few years, others exact no penalties for early repayment, and so on

Endowment mortgage
- Only interest is paid throughout the lifetime of the loan
- An endowment policy runs parallel with the loan and premiums are paid regularly (usually monthly)
- An endowment policy is a long-term regular (monthly) savings plan that also offers life insurance
- The policyholder's payments go into the insurance company's long-term investment fund, which, in turn, invests in a mixture of shares, government stock, company loans, property and other schemes
- At the end of the fixed period (usually 25 years) the loan is paid off from the proceeds
- At the end of the set period or if premature death occurs, the insurance company hands over a guaranteed lump sum called the 'sum assured'

Single account
- Your property is used as security for a borrowing facility that meets all personal financial needs; instead of separate accounts for mortgages, credit cards, current accounts or loans, one account covers all
- You agree a borrowing facility based on the value of your house and your annual income

continued...

Table 19 (continued)

Mortgages

- Your salary and any other income is paid into the single account
- You must stay within the agreed borrowing facility and repay the borrowings by the time you retire
- You must have life insurance to cover the borrowing facility at all times

it will be. Sickness insurance with the benefits deferred for 6 months should, for a 30-year-old, cost no more than £15 per month for £10 000 per annum until the age of 60.

Taxation

There is no point in paying more tax than you need to. Always submit details of tax-deductible expenses (e.g. professional and medical defence subscriptions) to the Inland Revenue; if there is a requirement to provide certain medical items, such as medical equipment, under the terms and conditions of employment in the NHS, submit a tax claim.

there is **no point** in **paying more tax** than you **need** to

Wills

Make a will with professional advice. Many individuals die intestate, leaving their relatives the potentially divisive task of guessing their intentions. You cannot assume that the law will follow your own logic when it comes to distributing your legacy.

Financial advisors

Most financial advisors are paid on a commission basis – the more they sell, the more commission they earn. Fully accredited independent financial advisors will offer their services on an hourly fee basis and return commissions. Always try to find an advisor who works independently. There are advisors who specialize in working with doctors – find out if your colleagues have any recommendations.

The middle years

With a consultant appointment comes your opportunity to move into private practice (see pages 57–69). Find yourself an accountant who specializes in advising doctors. He or she will advise you on the minutiae of accurate record-keeping and taxation issues.

Keeping records

It is essential that you regard your private practice as a business, and appreciate the need for accurate accounting records (Table 20) and regular reviews of income and expenditure.

Table 20
Finance in private practice

Organize
- A private practice bank account
- A separate credit card to cover incidental private practice expenditure (e.g. car and conference expenditure)

Keep
- A private practice petty-cash book that details practice cash expenditure (e.g. on stamps and small items of stationery)
- Full records of patient fees rendered
- The private practice patient appointments diary
- Accurate records of income and expenditure – complete the cheque book stubs and keep all invoices for expenditure (the law requires that all accounting records are maintained for a period of 6 years)

Private practice accounts have to be submitted to the Inland Revenue for taxation purposes annually; taxation is paid on the ultimate net profits. In addition to the normal running costs of the practice, tax relief is available on capital items of expenditure, such as cars, equipment, fixtures, fittings and furnishings. A sample profit and loss sheet is shown in Table 21.

Beware of the tax implications when undertaking private practice from your home. Be sure to take sound financial advice regarding this point. If your house is classified as a business rather than simply a residence, in theory, you may be liable for capital gains on its appreciation.

Pensions

NHS pension

It is worth considering investing in 'added years'. The NHS pension is calculated on length of service, each year of which counts as 1/80th of final salary. Most doctors qualify at 24 years of age and, at 60 years of age, would therefore receive a pension of 36/80ths of final salary. Additional years (called 'added years') to provide a pension of 40/80ths of final salary (i.e. half pay) can be purchased by additional monthly superannuation contributions of up to a maximum of 9% of salary.

> **'added years'** are an **excellent investment**

In terms of life expectancy, in order to recoup the 'added years' payment made during working life, you have to live up to 72.8 years of age. As most doctors can expect to live beyond this age, 'added years' are an excellent investment.

Personal pension

Over the years pension funding became increasingly complex, resulting in eight different regimes. On 6 April 2006 (A-Day), these were abolished and replaced with one single tax privilege regime. This regime is characterized as follows.

- There is a single lifetime allowance on the amount of pension savings that can benefit from tax relief.

Table 21

Sample private practice profit and loss account

		£	£
Income	Patient fees invoiced		125000
	Other fees (e.g. medicolegal)		4500
			129500
Expenses	Consulting room costs	9000	
	Secretary	15000	
	Drugs and medical purchases	1000	
	Assistants' fees	4000	
	Medical indemnity	9000	
	Printing, postage, stationery	750	
	Office costs (e.g. computer-related)	250	
	Books and journals	500	
	Bank charges and interest	800	
	Telephone in consulting rooms	300	
	Accountancy fees	1000	
	Bad debts	1500	
	Telephone and mobile phones (the proportion used on practice business)	500	
	Car expenses (practice proportion)	2500	
	Use of house for professional purposes	900	
	Spouse's assistance	3000	
	Spouse's pension contributions	1500	
	Conferences/courses (less refunds)	700	
	Depreciation	4200	
		56400	
Net profit for the year			**73100**

- The new lifetime limit every year will increase each year as follows:
  - 2006–07: £1.50 million
  - 2007–08: £1.60 million
  - 2008–09: £1.65 million
  - 2009–10: £1.75 million
  - 2010–11: £1.80 million

  and will then be reviewed and set for each subsequent 5-year period.
- The overall annual allowance of contributions for tax relief purposes is set at £215 000 for the 2006–07 tax year. It will be increased by £10 000/year for the next 4 tax years and then reviewed and set for the next 5 years.
- When the pension is taken after retirement, the fund will be tested against the limits; if the total exceeds the lifetime allowance, then if the funds are taken as a lump sum there will be a tax charge of 55% on the excess, and if they are taken as a pension there will be a tax charge of 25% on the excess, with the subsequent pension taxed at 40%.

Consultants who contribute to the NHS pension scheme and make further pension payments in respect of their private practices must take considerable care. Upon retirement, the fund value is calculated by multiplying the NHS pension by 20 and adding the tax-free lump sum, equivalent to 3 times the pension, to this figure (see the example in Table 22). For NHS consultants who will ultimately receive substantial merit awards, it is unlikely that there will be any scope for further private practice pension planning, and alternative investments should be considered.

The dos and don'ts of taxation

Complete the annual tax return form accurately and on time – failure to do this will automatically result in interest and penalties.

complete the **tax return on time**

Have a financial 'health check' from time to time – discuss your affairs with an accountant or tax advisor. Don't get caught without money in the bank when your tax bill arrives. Save for annual tax liabilities

Table 22

The pension of Mr White, Consultant Surgeon

Mr White has a substantial merit award, and has now completed 40 years of service, with a final salary of £130 000. Upon retirement, his pension entitlement will therefore be 40/80th his final salary, that is, half pay, £65 000, plus a tax-free lump sum of £195 000. The monetary value of Mr White's pension would be £65 000 × 20 = £1.3 million, plus the lump sum of £195 000, a total of £1.495 million. This figure is close to the new lifetime limit of £1.5 million, assuming Mr White retires in the year to 5 April 2007.

If Mr White has also been contributing to a personal pension and has accumulated funds of £300 000, at retirement this personal pension would be subject to the lifetime allowance charge of 55% if taken as a lump sum or, if taken as a pension, 25% on the excess with the subsequent pension being taxed at 40%.

However, two forms of protection of pension funds are available as at 5 April 2006.

If the lifetime allowance of £1.5 million has been exceeded at 5 April 2006, and no further pension payments are made, then no tax at the punitive rate of 55% will be payable when the pensions are taken. The reasoning behind this is that the pension funds were accumulated before the rules changed at 5 April 2006.

The other form of protection is called primary protection, whereby an individual who has exceeded the lifetime allowance of £1.5 million at April 2006 continues to make pension payments thereafter. If a doctor has a pension fund of £1.65 million at 5 April 2006, the fund is 10% above the lifetime allowance of £1.5 million. By choosing primary protection, whenever the doctor takes his/her pension, provided the value of the fund does not exceed 10% of the lifetime allowance at the date the pension is taken, then there would be no excess tax to pay. An individual has 3 years from 5 April 2006 to submit a protection of existing rights form to HM Revenue & Customs.

on a monthly basis; as a rough guide, set aside approximately one-third of your gross professional income.

Remember that tax legislation is subject to a review in the Chancellor's budget, and the law may change. Before you carry out any tax planning that will affect your situation in future years, ask yourself:

- how much the various forms of tax relief are worth to you
- how you could rearrange your affairs if the law was changed and the current forms of relief were curtailed or abolished.

Treat tax advice given over a gin and tonic sceptically. Very often friends or colleagues do not understand all the ramifications of their own tax affairs, let alone yours.

Be scrupulously honest and transparent about your financial affairs. Before you take any action, ask yourself whether you would be happy for all your tax affairs to be scrutinized by a tax inspector. Always account for all items of income and do not over-claim on expenses.

> would you be **happy** for all your affairs to be **scrutinized** by a **tax inspector?**

Retirement

For most people, this is the time of high net worth – your mortgage is, we hope, paid off, you may have moved to a smaller home and released capital, insurance policies may have matured and you may have inherited some money along the way. On average now, a man retiring at 60 will live for just over a further 21 years and a woman just over 25 years. These days, many doctors are retiring earlier, but early retirement must be planned for.

Recommendations

Take professional advice with regard to pension planning. Currently, there are so many different forms of pension on the market that you will benefit from an independent expert opinion. Your pension should be tailored to your personal circumstances. Also think about passing surplus capital down to your children or their children – this may save taxation in the form of death duties.

Consider the management of your investments. Investment decisions will vary according to the individual – factors will include:

- your age
- your income requirements
- the degree of risk that is acceptable to you
- expectations as to future levels of inflation
- perception of the economic climate.

In general terms, always ensure that when you are receiving a pension, your spouse is in receipt of the investment income, against which any personal tax allowances may be allocated.

Do not forget your will – does it need changing? Currently, inheritance tax is charged at a rate of 40% on all estates in excess of £285 000. In retirement, make use of annual exemptions whereby husband and wife can each give away £3000 in any tax year. If the full £3000 is not given in any year, the balance can be carried forward for 1 year only and is then allowable only if the exemption for the second year is used in full. Where an individual makes an irrevocable gift and survives for 7 years from the date of the gift, no inheritance tax is payable. If the donor does not survive for 7 years, the tax payable is reduced so that only a proportion is charged (Table 23). Always keep a record of gifts for possible scrutiny at a later date.

> try not to die as the **richest person** in the **graveyard**

Table 23
Timing of irrevocable gifts and inheritance tax

Years between gift and death	Tax payable (% of full amount due)
3–4	80
4–5	60
5–6	40
6–7	20

Avoiding the pitfalls

Be wary of passing on to younger generations so much capital that you may compromise your ability to pay for nursing home fees in the future.

Do not worry about spending appropriate amounts of capital in retirement if your pension does not allow you to maintain your standard of living.

Try not to die as the richest person in the graveyard – inheritance tax, currently at a rate of 40%, means that considerable amounts will have to be paid even after personal relief.

hiring and firing

Linky Trott LLB HONS
Edwin Coe Solicitors

*'Since my last report, this employee has
reached rock bottom and has started to dig'*
Extract from an appraisal

When you set up your private practice, you will almost certainly become
an employer, and you will need someone to manage your business. This
will be an entirely new role for most doctors and one for which you are
unlikely to be prepared. An increasing number of doctors are setting up in
partnerships, and there is a move towards the concept of chambers for
medical practitioners. This means that a practice may need to employ
more than one staff member in an administrative role, and therefore it is
all the more crucial that employment issues are properly addressed.

There is a wealth of information available on the basic nuts and bolts
of employees' entitlements such as pay, working time, maternity leave and
so on, which you can find in the Employment Relations section of the
Department of Trade and Industry (DTI) website (http://www.dti.gov.
uk/er/). Practical advice on the employment relationship is, however, less
readily available, as is guidance on the common pitfalls that can make the
relationship go sour and can be expensive.

Choosing the right person

The role of the doctor's wife as practice manager or as part-time
secretary/bookkeeper is a time-honoured one which suits some
consultants; unfortunately, though, women doctors whose husbands
perform this role are few and far between. The arrangement is certainly

worth looking at, because you will not find anyone quite as motivated as your spouse to see that your fees are paid! In addition, there are tax advantages in having your partner on the payroll of the business, and you should explore these with your accountant.

> there are **tax advantages** in having your **partner** on the **payroll**

While you may have some say in the recruitment of secretaries at your NHS practice, the recruitment is likely to be orchestrated by the personnel department. For your private work, you are on your own. If you are not fortunate enough to have a spouse as practice manager, it is vital that you remember these three things.

- You must take care to make the right choice in the first place, not settling for second best just because there seems to be nobody much else around and you are keen to get on as soon as possible.
- You must be aware of your obligations as an employer.
- You must know how to tackle problems when they arise, so that you don't end up facing an employment tribunal with thousands of pounds to pay in compensation.

Recruitment and staff contracts

You may already know someone who would like to work for you, or you may need to advertise. Either way, it is important to prepare a job description and a person specification against which you can measure the candidates' qualifications, experience and personality. Note that there must be no discrimination when preparing the job advertisement, selecting which candidates to interview, assessing candidates at interview or at any time during their employment. 'Discrimination' includes sex, race and disability discrimination, of course, but less obviously includes discrimination on the grounds of religion, sexual orientation and age (as against the young and the old).

Be meticulous about taking up references, speaking personally to as many previous employers as possible; and don't be afraid to probe deeper if you sense that the referee is in any way hesitant or if you think there is something to be read between the lines.

You are obliged to provide certain information to a new employee within 8 weeks of their starting date. This written statement should cover the main terms of employment, which are summarized in Table 24;

be **meticulous** about taking up **references**

a full list can be found on the DTI's website. Build a probationary period into the contract (usually 3 to 6 months) during which there is a relatively short notice period of a week. This should give you time to decide whether the relationship is going to work.

Good employment practice

The key to good employment practice is to deal with issues as they arise and record them. If your secretary is persistently late, for example, you must start tackling this directly early on.

Table 24

Statement of main terms of employment

- Names of the parties
- Date employment began and statement about any continuity recognized
- Job title and/or brief description of the work
- Place of work
- Salary and other benefits including intervals of payment
- Hours of work
- Holiday entitlement (minimum 4 weeks)
- Sick pay and sick leave arrangements
- Pension arrangements (if none, this must be stated); whether there is a contracting out certificate in force
- Period of notice or length of contract
- Details of any collective agreements affecting the employment (if none, this must be stated)
- Grievance, disciplinary and appeals procedure (or reference to these)

Annual performance appraisals should be held to address strengths and weaknesses, and all comments from both sides should be documented and kept on the employee's personnel file. Review any goals set at the previous year's appraisal, and do not shy away from difficult confrontational issues, such as an unhelpful attitude. An appraisal is not the same thing as a disciplinary hearing, however; if misdemeanours are raised at an appraisal, do not think that this will count as formal disciplinary action.

an **appraisal** is not a **disciplinary hearing**

When things go wrong

It may seem a little perverse to dwell on the degeneration of the employment relationship, but if you are aware of the potential problems you could save yourself a considerable amount of time, anxiety and money. The first thing to note is that an employee can bring a claim against their employer without leaving the employment. Do not think, therefore, that if you haven't actually dismissed them they don't have a claim.

Claims can be brought against you for a broad range of issues, the most common of which are: unfair dismissal; wrongful dismissal or breach of contract; discrimination on the grounds of sex, race or disability; unfair selection for redundancy and unlawful deductions from wages. Unfair dismissal is by far the most common claim brought to an employment tribunal, so it is worth being aware of the main issues.

unfair dismissal is **the most common** claim

An employee cannot claim unfair dismissal until he or she has been in post for 1 year. In calculating this, a Tribunal will add the statutory notice period of 1 week. Five specific reasons for dismissal are defined in the Employment Rights Act 1966, and employees can be dismissed only for one of these reasons. The most important are:

- shortcomings in the capability or qualifications of the employee
- misconduct of the employee
- redundancy.

Clearly, the dismissal of any employee on the grounds of misconduct or capability is a process that must be developed over a period of time, and there is a statutory obligation to go through a formal disciplinary or dismissal procedure. This is referred to as the 'letter, meeting, appeal' procedure and is described in more detail below.

Capability issues

When new systems, procedures or equipment are introduced, existing staff are likely to have difficulties and will need specific training. If you have taken all reasonable measures to help them and they still have difficulty, they should be given clear and ample warning to improve. Document any discussions on the subject – a tribunal will be more inclined to sympathize with you if there is evidence that you consulted

> **follow** the formal **'letter, meeting, appeal'** procedure at every stage

your employee and considered any suggestions they have. You should follow the formal 'letter, meeting, appeal' procedure at every stage save for the first informal discussion.

Misconduct issues

Gross misconduct (e.g. stealing from petty cash) may justify dismissal without notice, but lesser misdemeanours, ranging from the merely irritating to the outright insupportable, will have to be handled carefully, and every stage must be covered by the 'letter, meeting, appeal' procedure.

If your secretary is consistently late in the mornings, for example, a reasonable first step would be to hold an informal meeting to discuss the reasons for this. If the secretary explains that the trains are always late, you could discuss alternatives such as trying to catch an earlier train or altering their hours to start half an hour later in the morning and finish later in the evening. This serves a number of purposes.

- It demonstrates that you are a 'reasonable' employer in the event that the problem escalates and you end up before an employment tribunal.

- It sends an important message to the secretary that 'swinging the lead' will not be tolerated in your practice.

If the secretary continues to be late or other conduct issues arise, such as taking long lunch hours or leaving early, you should begin the formal 'letter, meeting, appeal' process. The 'letter' is a requirement to set out in writing the conduct complained of or the other circumstances that give rise to consideration of disciplinary sanctions or dismissal. The letter should notify the relevant individual of the following in writing:

- the conduct complained of, together with any supporting evidence
- the fact that you consider this to be a formal disciplinary matter
- confirmation that no conclusions will be drawn until you have heard the employee's representations
- the fact that you are calling a formal disciplinary meeting to discuss the issue and hear explanations
- when the hearing will take place
- the types of sanctions you are considering if, after the meeting, you consider the misconduct to have been substantiated; these may include an oral warning, a formal written warning and dismissal, either with or without notice
- the fact that the employee has a right to be accompanied to the hearing by a work colleague or union representative.

Following the disciplinary meeting you should consider the appropriate sanction and notify the employee of their right to appeal and the fact that they may be accompanied to the appeal by a colleague or union representative. If they wish to appeal you should hold an appeal meeting. Dismissal is unlikely to be a 'reasonable' approach for a first misdemeanour. It may be appropriate to note an oral or written warning on the personnel file for a period of 1 year. If there are any further transgressions, the same procedure should be adopted as before to allow the employee to give any relevant explanations (e.g. absence as a result of a death in the family would not justify going on to the next disciplinary stage).

One of the most difficult and frustrating areas to deal with is the employee who seems constantly to be 'off sick'. You must be seen to have acted reasonably in treating the ill-health of an employee as a

> **notify** the employee of their **right to appeal**

reason to dismiss (either as a conduct issue for bad attendance, as a capability issue due to sickness, or for some other substantial reason). You will also have to consider whether or not the sickness indicates an underlying disability for which accommodation should be made. You can arm yourself well in advance by including the following items in the contract of employment:

- a clause detailing how long the employee will be paid normal salary when he or she is off work on the grounds of ill-health; commonly there is a provision that the employee will be paid normal salary for an aggregate of 4 weeks out of every rolling 12-month period and thereafter will receive statutory sick pay only
- a clause requiring employees who are absent on the grounds of ill-health to complete a self-certification form in respect of each day of absence and to provide a doctor's certificate on the fourth consecutive day of any absence; this will enable you to keep a proper record of sickness that can act as an independent record of ill-health absences if required.

Long-term sickness absence requires full consultation and communication with the employee, and a tribunal will want to be satisfied that you have acquainted yourself with all the relevant facts before instigating any disciplinary action. You may, for example, ask the employee's GP for the short, medium and long-term prognosis. You should also be able to demonstrate that you did consider reasonable adjustments to the type or hours of work, or any other suggestions made by the employee or their GP, and you should make it clear that you are taking decisions for employment, not medical reasons. Detailed consideration of the procedure to adopt where an employee is off on long-term sickness absence is outside the scope of this chapter, but given the possible application of the Disability Discrimination Act in these circumstances, it would be prudent to take advice from an employment lawyer before taking any disciplinary action or dismissing.

> long-term sickness absence requires full consultation and communication

You may gain some comfort from the fact that, for the small employer, tribunals will consider the impact of the employee's absence on colleagues and the effect on their workload, as well as on the business in general.

Redundancies

It is not an easy option to dismiss an employee on the grounds of redundancy, and it is only really possible if you have at least one other employee. Remember also that only roles, not people, are redundant, although obviously the redundancy of a role can affect an employee's continued employment. The employee may dispute that there was a true redundancy situation, and may challenge you on whether you acted fairly in selecting them for redundancy and not one of your other employees. You must ask yourself the following questions.

- Is there a true redundancy situation (i.e. do you require fewer people to undertake the same amount of work)? If so, the tribunal will ask you why. If it is because there is a downturn in business, you will have to demonstrate that. For instance, you may have bought a bookkeeping software package and you propose to ask your secretary to run this from her system, thereby making redundant the role of the other employee who does the bookkeeping.

- What objective criteria must you apply to decide who will be selected for redundancy? 'Last in, first out' was traditionally the most objective selection criterion, but is likely to be discriminatory on the grounds of age. Tribunals appreciate that it is necessary to look at your requirements, and will expect a consideration of a number of objective selection criteria, which could include cost, qualifications, disciplinary record etc.

To continue with the above example, you are likely to assess that you will require someone who is capable of typing complex medical reports and running bookkeeping software on your office computer system. Your current secretary would score more favourably and the bookkeeper is therefore 'at risk' of redundancy. You must send the bookkeeper the letter referred to above as part of the 'letter, meeting, appeal' process and state that you propose to enter into a period of consultation during which you would like them to make suggestions as to how a redundancy may be avoided. The bookkeeper may suggest, for example, that they are familiar with that software and would

the **consultation** process must include a **meeting**

be happy to work just 1 day a week. This may suit your purposes, but would never have been known if you had not undergone a consultation period. The consultation process must include at least one meeting, as required in the 'letter, meeting, appeal' process.

Following a short consultation period, you should then make a final decision and issue your notice of dismissal on the grounds of redundancy, advising the employee of their right to appeal. You should continue to consider the redeployment of the affected staff member to a different role in your business for the duration of any notice period. If, for example, you were thinking of retaining a researcher at the same time, you should consider your bookkeeper for the role. If you don't consult, you won't know if the individual has any research experience or interest. You are, of course, entitled to consider them in the same way as you would assess any other candidate for the job.

Constructive dismissal

In order to lodge a claim for unfair dismissal before an employment tribunal, an employee must demonstrate that they have been dismissed. Obviously, if you tell your secretary to leave and take her annoying, tedious little habits with her and never return, that will amount to a dismissal. Under some circumstances, however, a tribunal will find that although you have not actually dismissed your employee, they will consider it so because you have breached a fundamental term of the employment contract. This could arise if you decided to reduce an employee's salary without their consent (not likely to be given!); less obviously, it could arise if you breach a term implicit in all contracts of employment to the effect that both parties will demonstrate a sufficient degree of mutual trust and confidence in each other. This is considered fundamental to the contract, and you can find yourself in breach of it if, for example, you consistently bully (or allow another individual to bully) an employee. So, if you frequently reduce your secretary to tears, beware! You may find that she leaves you and lodges a claim for unfair constructive dismissal.

If an employee raises a grievance with you in writing at any time, you must call a meeting with them to discuss it, notify them of your findings in connection with their grievance and give them a right to appeal against that finding at a further meeting.

Getting help

It is a sound rule of thumb that prevention is better than cure, and this is certainly true when it comes to employment relations. Make sure you communicate and consult with your employees and keep them fully informed of business decisions that may affect them. Whether hiring or firing, do not take the well-meant advice of friends and colleagues, but get proper professional help. Half an hour spent with an experienced employment lawyer can save a great deal of unpleasantness when you find yourself in the unenviable position of having 'trouble with the staff'.

Further reading and resources

Advisory, Conciliation and Arbitration Service (ACAS)
http://www.acas.org.uk

Department of Trade and Industry
http://www.dti.gov.uk/er/

medicolegal matters

Dr Michael Devlin
Medical Defence Union

*'The Common Law of England has been laboriously built about a
mythical figure – the figure of "The Reasonable Man"'*
Uncommon Law, AP Herbert (1935)

There is a very important overlap between the disciplines of medicine,
ethics and the law. Indeed, this is recognized by the General Medical
Council (GMC) in its guidance to medical undergraduates. The guidance in
Tomorrow's Doctors states that graduates must know about and
understand the main ethical and legal issues they will come across. This
includes an understanding of confidentiality, of how to respond to
patients' complaints and also of how to deal with problems in the
performance, conduct or health of colleagues. The GMC also emphasizes
that graduates must understand the principles and good practice of
obtaining consent from patients. Many doctors will have a good
understanding of ethicolegal principles in medicine, and the aim of this
chapter is to assist in reinforcing those principles.

In this brief summary I can give only a flavour of some practical
aspects of medicolegal principles. I hope that readers will not be too
dismayed at the legal processes they might face in the future. The concept
of 'multiple jeopardy' is with us, in the sense that, as a result of a single
incident, a doctor may face NHS complaint, inquest civil claim, criminal
investigation and referral to the GMC. However, most medicine is
practised to a good standard and is coupled with consistent and
reasonable application of legal and ethical principles. Perhaps the most
useful advice I can give to a junior doctor starting out in hospital
medicine is to be familiar with the GMC's guidance in *Good Medical
Practice*. That document sets out the standards that are expected of a

professionally qualified, registered medical practitioner, and it is incumbent upon all doctors to be thoroughly familiar with the content.

'*The evil that men do lives after them, the good is oft interred with their bones*'. When one peruses media reports, Shakespeare's words sometimes appear prophetic. Medical mishaps feature prominently in reports about the profession. However, most contacts doctors have with their patients result in positive outcomes rather than a complaint or claim, and media reports should be read in this context.

Patient rights

There can be little doubt that the emphasis in the doctor–patient relationship has changed over time. Whereas medical paternalism might have been part of normal practice throughout much of the early twentieth century, there is little doubt that it would find no favour in today's society. To students of ethical principles this should come as no surprise: the principle of autonomy predicates patients' rights to self-determination. The greater profile of patients' rights and their contribution to the way the NHS functions is recognized in statute (the Health and Social Care Act 2001), a purpose of which is, inter alia, '...*to strengthen the way the public and patients are involved in the way the NHS works.*' Doctors pursuing a career in hospital medicine will wish to ensure that they actively involve their patients in decisions that affect the patients.

Confidentiality

a **patient** must be **sure** that a **doctor** will **treat** anything occurring in a professional setting as **confidential**

Arguably the duty of confidence is at the very heart of the doctor–patient relationship. That relationship must be founded on mutual trust and respect, and in consequence a patient must be sure that a doctor will treat and respect anything occurring in a professional setting as confidential.

Essentially, confidentiality is governed by ethical principles, by the common-law duty of confidence and by statute (in particular the Data Protection Act 1998). The ethical principles of confidentiality are set out in the GMC publication *Confidentiality: Protecting and Providing Information*. The GMC's guidance is detailed, and doctors must be familiar with it, since a failure to follow the guidance may put their registration at risk. The guidance is easily accessible from the GMC's website (http://www.gmc-uk.org) if you should find yourself having to consider details of it while you are at work. The GMC states, for example:

Doctors hold information about patients which is private and sensitive. This information must not be given to others unless the patient consents or you can justify the disclosure.

When you are satisfied that information should be released, you should act promptly to disclose all relevant information. This is often essential to the best interests of the patient, or to safeguard the well-being of others.

A question might arise as to what precisely constitutes confidential information. A useful working definition is that any information that you possess about a patient solely because of your professional relationship with the patient must be considered to be confidential. This includes, for example, the mere fact that the patient is under your care and also includes the patient's biographical details held on file. Confidential information will certainly include medical details of their illnesses and treatment.

> **disclosure** can be made **with the consent of the patient**

The GMC's guidance explains how confidential information can be lawfully disclosed in essentially one of two ways. Firstly, disclosure can be made with the consent of the patient. The patient is presumed in law to have capacity (competence; see the section on consent later in this chapter), but in some patients it may be necessary to formally assess capacity.

The second set of circumstances in which confidential information about a patient may be disclosed to a third party, even without consent, is where disclosure is required by law, such as notification of certain communicable diseases and notification to the police required by the Terrorism Act 2000, or where the public interest in disclosure outweighs the patient's own interest in confidentiality. The GMC's guidance states that the public interest is likely to prevail, for example, where a failure to disclose information may expose the patient or others to risk of death or serious harm. The guidance goes on to state that such situations might arise where disclosure may assist in the prevention, detection or prosecution of a serious crime, particularly crimes against the person (such as abuse of children).

The consequences of breaching confidence unlawfully include the possibilities that the patient might pursue a doctor (or the NHS Trust that employs the doctor) in the civil courts, might complain to the GMC or might make a complaint to the Information Commissioner in respect of a breach of the Data Protection Act 1998. Consequently, any particularly difficult decisions as regards whether or not to disclose information to a third party (for example, the police) should be discussed with a senior and experienced colleague and with your medical defence organization.

The patient's right to confidentiality is also protected by the European Convention on Human Rights under Article 8 (incorporated into domestic law by virtue of the Human Rights Act 1998). Remaining on the topic of European jurisprudence, the Data Protection Act 1998 (DPA) gives legal effect to a European Directive on personal data (European Parliament and Council Directive 95/46/EC). The DPA essentially regulates the processing of personal information about living individuals and includes the obtaining, use of or disclosure of that information. It does not apply to deceased individuals. It applies to both paper and electronic records.

Patients, in the terminology of the DPA, are 'data subjects' and they have certain rights:

- to be told that data is held about them and of the purposes for which their data will be processed
- to have access to the data
- to have data corrected when it is inaccurate.

For the purposes of hospital practice, the question that is most likely to arise is whether the patient can have access to their clinical records (a question usually arising from a subject access request by the patient). In the majority of cases this will be straightforward and the information will simply be disclosed. However, the Act does give certain exemptions, including what might be called 'therapeutic privilege'. In the exercise of therapeutic privilege, a doctor may decide that information should not be disclosed if it would be likely to cause serious harm to the patient's physical or mental health (or to the physical or mental health of another individual). Information identifying a third party who is not a healthcare professional can be exempted under the Act if certain requirements are met. Specific information relating to the application of the Data Protection Act can be found in a publication by the Information Commissioner entitled *Use and disclosure of health data*. However, particular problems may arise in respect of children, adults without capacity and the deceased. It is useful briefly to touch upon these three groups.

Children

Once they have attained the age of 16 (see the section on Consent and children later in this chapter), children are entitled to consent to medical treatment. Consequently, they are entitled to the same confidentiality as an adult patient. The situation pertaining to children aged 15 years and under is less straightforward because parental involvement is usual and brings with it the sharing of knowledge about the child with the parents. However, in any decision concerning the divulging of a child's

> **children** of sufficient maturity have **the same right** to **confidentiality** as an adult

information the principal consideration must be that the decision to disclose must always be in the best interests of the child. Additionally, consideration must be given to whether the child has capacity to consent to the disclosure. If a child is 'Gillick competent' (has sufficient maturity and understanding of what is involved in the proposed treatment or disclosure) then he or she also has a right to exercise consent about what is disclosed. In accordance with the judgment of Lord Fraser in the *Gillick* case (Table 25), where a child does not want to divulge information, it is important that every effort must be made to persuade the child to involve their parents or guardians.

Where a child (including those children up to 18 years) is not competent to give consent, a parent or someone with parental responsibility must provide authority to disclose confidential information on the child's behalf. (Parental responsibility is a legal status derived from the Children Act 1989.) The married parents of the child will automatically have parental responsibility, as will the mother, irrespective of whether the parents were married. An unmarried father may acquire parental responsibility if he becomes registered as the child's father and his name subsequently appears on the child's birth certificate from December 2003, or where there is a formal agreement with the child's mother, or where a court order confers on him parental responsibility. In some circumstances, such as when a child is taken into care, the local authority may have parental responsibility. It is also possible for a court to remove parental responsibility.

Adults with incapacity

This category applies to those over 18 years of age. It is important not to make an automatic presumption of lack of capacity in patients who have mental disorders or learning disabilities. The law provides for a rebuttable presumption of capacity in all adults (see also the section later in this chapter on the criteria for judging capacity, page 167). In England and Wales, at present, nobody can make treatment decisions for a patient who is an incompetent adult, and such decisions are made by those providing clinical care to the patient in accordance with their best interests. Generally speaking, the same applies to disclosure of confidential information. Disclosure should normally only be made to a third party where the clinician believes it is in the patient's best interests.

Often a doctor will want to share information with relatives or friends of the patient. If the patient is unable to consent, disclosure can be made so long as it is in the patient's best interests to do so.

> there is a rebuttable
> **presumption of capacity in all adults**

The Mental Capacity Act 2005 provides for an independent mental capacity advocate for patients who lack capacity and who do not have anyone to authorize treatment on their behalf; these advocates will come into being from 2007 when the Act becomes operative. Consequently, decisions about disclosure are likely to be considered by the advocate on behalf of the patient at that time. In Scotland, the Adults with Incapacity (Scotland) Act 2000 allows welfare attorneys (and other 'proxy decision-makers') to be appointed when a patient lacks capacity. Decisions about disclosure should be discussed with the welfare attorney as and when the need arises.

Deceased patients

The GMC's guidance on confidentiality makes it clear that the duty of confidence persists after death. Where a patient has died and a third party requests disclosure of confidential information, then authority should be sought from the patient's personal representatives (normally the executor or other person responsible for the administration of the estate). Any views expressed by the patient before death must be respected. Disclosures after a patient's death

> the **duty of confidence** persists after **death**

are also governed by statute (Access to Health Records Act 1990), which provides that anyone who may have a claim arising out of a patient's death may be entitled to apply to have access to the patient's clinical records.

Consent

As stated earlier, it is the principle of autonomy that defines a patient's ethical right to decide what happens to them. It is essential that a doctor has the patient's consent before examination or providing treatment; failure to do so may result in a criminal investigation, a civil claim or a complaint to the GMC. The GMC has published detailed guidance (*Seeking Patients' Consent: The Ethical Considerations*), which sets out the ethicolegal basis of consent. In particular, the GMC emphasizes that doctors must obtain valid consent. In order to be valid, it must be informed. In other words, patients *must* be given enough information to make an informed choice about whether to accept the treatment. Consent may then be implied or expressed, but doctors should get the patient's express consent for any procedures that carry significant risk. This means that the patient must clearly express his or her consent to the particular treatment. Express consent may be oral or written, but it is usual to get written consent signed by the patient for major procedures. Where consent is oral a clear note must be made to record it.

> doctors must **obtain**
> **informed consent**

The timing in obtaining consent can be important. It goes without saying that patient's consent, for example to a surgical procedure, should be obtained before the start of the procedure and before the patient is sedated. It may be prudent to obtain the patient's consent at an outpatient clinic well in advance of the procedure itself and then to allow the patient to reaffirm their consent when they are admitted for the procedure proper. For practical purposes, the person who discusses the procedure with the patient should, whenever possible, be the individual who carries out that procedure. Where that is not possible, the task of obtaining consent should only be delegated to someone who is suitably trained and qualified, has sufficient knowledge of the proposed treatment and understands the risks involved.

Another aspect of valid consent is that it must be given freely by the patient and be devoid of any untoward external influence or duress. For example, in *Re T* an adult's refusal of treatment that was necessary to save life was invalid because of duress exerted by the patient's mother.

Competence (capacity)

Another feature of valid consent is that it must be given by a competent person. The legal criteria for competence were set out in the case of *Re C*, where a patient with schizophrenia refused treatment for a gangrenous leg. The court held that the patient had capacity to decide whether or not to accept a doctor's advice regarding treatment, notwithstanding any concurrent mental illness. The criteria for competence were set out as follows.

- The patient must comprehend and retain information provided regarding treatment.
- The patient must believe the information given.
- The patient must be able to weigh in the balance what they have been told in order to arrive at a choice.

For practical purposes, guidance published jointly by the BMA and the Law Society states that in order to demonstrate capacity

Individuals should be able to:

- *understand in simple language what the medical treatment is, its nature and purpose, and why it is being proposed*
- *understand its principal benefits, risks and alternatives*
- *understand in broad terms what will be the consequences of not receiving the proposed treatment*
- *retain the information for long enough to use it and weigh it in the balance in order to arrive at a decision.*

It should be noted that for adult patients there is a presumption of capacity. In other words, a doctor should approach a patient assuming that they have capacity to decide on treatment and it is only in cases where it can be demonstrated that the patient does not have capacity that treatment, if necessary, may be given in the absence of consent. A further important point to bear in mind is that the degree of capacity required to deal with decisions might vary, depending on what the nature

> **for adult patients** there is a **presumption** of **capacity**

of that decision is. Therefore, an individual with impaired capacity may have capacity to decide whether or not to accept treatment for a benign skin lesion, but may not be able to weigh in the balance more complex decisions to be made concerning treatment for a serious medical condition that might ultimately bring about their death. Where a patient does have capacity to decide on treatment, this includes decisions to refuse treatment. If there is ever any doubt about capacity then it is worthwhile asking a senior colleague (or other specialist) to assist in the evaluation of the patient.

Advance directives

Advance directives, if properly executed, are lawful and may be binding upon medical staff. The advance directive should clearly set out the circumstances under which the patient either wishes for treatment or refuses it. The advance refusal of treatment would be binding on the patient's doctors where the presenting circumstances were those envisaged when the consent was given. However, advance consent to treatment would only be binding on the treating doctors where they felt it was in the patient's best interests. This can occasionally cause difficulties where the directive is written in vague terms, and it may be necessary to seek advice from your medical defence organization or your hospital's legal advisors in doubtful cases.

Treatment of incompetent adults

Difficulties potentially arise in circumstances where an adult patient is incapable of consenting to treatment. In such situations, treatment of the patient can be given lawfully under common-law principles. This means that treatment can be provided to an incompetent patient if it is in their best interests. The term 'best interests' has a wider meaning than simply what is in the patient's best medical interests. It should reflect a holistic assessment of the patient's situation, and doctors are advised to consult as widely as possible in relation to it. This may include seeking the views of relatives and carers, the patient's GP and other individuals who might have an interest in the patient's welfare. However, it is ultimately for the treating doctor to make a decision as to what is in the patient's

treatment may be given in the patient's **best interests** where there is **temporary incapacity**

best interests and provide treatment accordingly. An adult relative cannot 'consent' on behalf of an incompetent patient, although where there is disagreement between the relatives and the doctors, it is wise to seek legal advice, and in such situations the conflict may need to be put before the court. Also, in rare circumstances there may be some doubt as to the reliability of the assessment of capacity, or concerns that proposed treatment might be non-therapeutic. It is therefore sometimes necessary to apply to the High Court under its inherent jurisdiction to obtain a declaration that what is proposed in respect of the patient is concerned is lawful. It is likely that the trust's solicitors would be involved in any such application to the High Court.

Treatment may also be given in the patient's best interests where there is temporary incapacity, but where the treatment is necessary immediately to save life or avoid significant deterioration in the patient's health. This situation often arises in emergencies, such as a patient who is incapable owing to unconsciousness after a car accident but who requires urgent treatment. In such circumstances treatment may be justified under the common-law doctrine of necessity. This duty to treat under the doctrine of necessity was set out by Lord Brandon in *Re F*.

For reasons of space, I do not propose to deal here with the Mental Health Act 1983, which is currently being amended, and the treatments of mental disorders. Where there is any doubt about treatment to be provided to a patient for their mental illness then advice should be sought from an appropriate professional source such as a medical defence organization.

Consent and children

The Family Law Reform Act 1969, Section 8(1), provides that the legal age for consent for medical, surgical and dental treatment is 16 years and over. The law is not so clear-cut in relation to a young person's decision to refuse treatment, even if they are over the age of 16. In *Re W* the Court of Appeal held that the parents of a child who was 16 or 17 could authorize treatment for them – the minor had no legal right of veto. Any treatment provided to children must be in their best interests. However, it is hoped that such situations will be exceptional, and in circumstances where a competent 16- or 17-year-old child refuses treatment that is advised, it would be prudent to seek appropriate medicolegal advice.

Children under the age of 16 may, under common-law principles, consent to treatment. The matter was considered by the courts in 1985 and ultimately went to the House of Lords in the case of *Gillick*.

The starting point in deciding whether to treat a 'Gillick-competent' child is to seek to persuade them to involve their parents in the decision. Lord Fraser in *Gillick* set out some guidance where, in relation to providing contraceptive treatment, a doctor would be justified in proceeding without parental consent or knowledge in circumstances where a child refused to involve their parents:

- the child, although less than 16 years of age, understands the doctor's advice; and
- the doctor cannot persuade the child to inform their parents regarding the matter; and (in the particular case, which concerned provision of contraception to a girl)
- the child was likely to begin or continue having sexual intercourse with or without contraceptive treatment; and
- unless the child received contraceptive advice or treatment her physical or mental health, or both, were likely to suffer; and
- the child's best interests required the doctor to give her contraceptive advice, treatment or both without parental consent.

Although this case was concerned with the provision of contraceptive advice to girls, it has application to other medical or surgical treatments. Children under 16 years of age can only consent to treatment where they understand its nature, purpose and hazards. The 'nature' of the procedure is very important as the child's understanding may vary depending on the complexity of the treatment proposed. There is no particular age at which a child under 16 will be able to consent to treatment: one might be dealing with an immature child who is a day away from their sixteenth birthday or a mature child who is only 10. The assessment of capacity needs to be made on an individual basis and for an individual proposal of treatment or examination; it is a question of fact in each case.

there is **no particular age** at which a **child** under 16 will be able to **consent to treatment**

Within the confines of this chapter, it is not possible to go into much detail on this highly complex area of law and ethics.

Regulation and discipline of doctors

It is difficult to approach hospital medicine without at least some knowledge of what might happen when things go wrong. This is important, because seeking professional help at the outset might be crucial in determining an appropriate outcome.

NHS complaints procedure and clinical governance

Although few doctors will experience disciplinary proceedings or investigation by the GMC, most will experience the relatively common occurrence of a complaint at least once in their careers. The NHS Complaints Procedure has three distinct parts:

- local resolution (where the matter, in the case of NHS Hospitals, is dealt with by the hospital trust, and an explanation provided to the patient in writing)
- independent review (where the case is reviewed or investigated by the Healthcare Commission)
- the Health Service Ombudsman.

Upon receipt of a complaint, a doctor would need carefully to review the clinical records in order to provide an explanation. If appropriate, an apology should be given; this does not equate to an admission of liability. The local resolution phase of the NHS complaints procedure may involve a certain amount of dovetailing with clinical governance procedures. Therefore, there might be also an investigation into what went wrong in order to establish whether there could be improvements to procedures to prevent a recurrence.

Doctors should cooperate with any such investigation into their (or a colleague's) conduct, performance or health. This obligation to cooperate with enquiries is set out in the GMC's publication *Good Medical Practice*.

cooperate with any **investigation** into **conduct, performance or health**

Hospital discipline

Within the NHS, procedures exist for the initial handling of concerns about doctors and dentists. The framework document is known as *Maintaining High Professional Standards in the Modern NHS*. A detailed account of the procedures is beyond the scope of this chapter, but suffice it to say that the framework provides for procedures whereby concerns about a doctor's conduct or performance are initially investigated and a decision then taken as to whether to proceed with a formal disciplinary hearing (under Part 3 of the document). There are separate procedures for dealing with problems of professional performance (capability) and for dealing with a doctor's health problems. The framework document also sets out how a doctor might need to be suspended from duties whilst an investigation takes place (this is now known as 'exclusion').

Disciplinary procedures are both daunting and stressful and it is vital to make contact with your medical defence organization at the outset.

The General Medical Council

The GMC has various functions, including a requirement to maintain a register of medical practitioners, and in the case of hospital doctors, a Specialist Register as well. The GMC has statutory powers to deal with doctors whose fitness to practise may be impaired. Such impairment of fitness to practise can arise, in the main, because of issues of misconduct, poor performance or ill health (other circumstances also apply, such as convictions and adverse findings by other registration bodies).

The GMC's procedures provide for an initial investigatory phase, which is usually dealt with by way of written submissions, and a second adjudication phase in which allegations of impairment to fitness to practise are considered by a Fitness to Practise Panel. At such hearings, fitness to practise is considered 'in the round' which means the panel can consider concerns about misconduct, health and poor performance at the same time. The Fitness to Practise Panel, having heard the evidence, will decide whether or not the doctor's fitness to practise is impaired and, if there is impairment, decide upon appropriate sanction. The GMC follows its indicative sanctions guidance in deciding what penalty to impose upon a doctor's registration, and this can range from striking a doctor from the register (erasure) to conditions on registration. Additionally, where fitness to practise is not impaired, a panel may nonetheless issue a warning where there has been a significant departure from good medical practice or a significant cause for concern following assessment of a doctor's performance.

Civil litigation

At the outset of this chapter, mention was made of the reasonable man; the significance of that quotation will perhaps become more apparent on reading this section. Doctors working in the NHS and elsewhere are under a duty to attend their patients with due care and attention, using reasonable skill. Patients are entitled to sue when they suffer financially compensatable harm as a result of the hospital's negligence. This type of legal action is known as tort, and in the case of claims against the NHS will arise from allegations of clinical negligence. Such civil litigation is not intended to be punitive. Financial awards of compensation are not made to punish a particular trust or clinician: they are made to put the patient back in the position in which they would have been had it not been for the negligence causing injury. For a claim to succeed, a claimant must show:

- that a duty of care was owed to them; and
- that there was a breach in that duty of care (negligence); and
- that the negligence caused the injury that is the basis of the claim.

Once a patient has been accepted for treatment by a hospital trust then a duty of care arises. The test for professional negligence is set out in the classic case of *Bolam*. In essence, the test is that a medical practitioner is not negligent if they act in accordance with a responsible and respectable body of medical opinion skilled in that particular art. A doctor is also judged by the standards of their peers in that particular specialty and also by the standards of the day when treatment was provided. Reasonableness, in relation to the standard of care, will largely reflect usual and accepted

> **civil litigation** is **not** intended to be **punitive**

practice, and the court will usually be informed by expert opinion in that regard. However, reasonableness by reference to a responsible and respectable body of medical opinion is not absolute. As was made clear in the case of *Bolitho*, the body of medical opinion must be capable of withstanding logical analysis: the court is the final arbiter of what is reasonable.

Within the NHS, hospital trusts are vicariously liable for the acts and omissions of their employees. Consequently, clinical negligence claims are normally brought against trusts rather than individual medical practitioners, and therefore trusts' litigation services managers, lawyers or the NHS Litigation Authority will deal with claims that arise from the provision of care to NHS patients.

Hospital doctors' involvement in the process is likely to be in providing witness statements to the trust's lawyers or the NHS Litigation Authority. The provision of such statements should concentrate on detailing a doctor's factual involvement in their attendance upon the patient.

Tort of breach of statutory duty

Health and safety prosecutions, although rare, can occur where patients or staff have been injured, or they have suffered severe health problems (e.g. stress or a latex-allergy-related illness) and the trust did not have suitable policies in place to prevent that damage.

Trusts can be sued for the tort of Breach of Statutory Duty where their failure to comply with health and safety law has resulted in an employee or patients suffering a work-related injury. Since 2003, injured employees could also sue the trust if it has failed to adequately assess the risks to their health and safety at work.

Criminal matters

It is necessary in this chapter, for completeness, to say a word or two about potential criminal liability for serious criminal or health and safety offences, but it is very rare for a doctor to be involved in a criminal investigation related to their clinical care of patients. The two main types of criminal investigations that doctors may find themselves facing as a result of their professional clinical practice are allegations of homicide or of assault (including sexual assault.)

Homicide

Most homicide cases will be prosecuted as gross negligence manslaughter, although a certain number of cases have been prosecuted over the years in which doctors are alleged to have murdered their patients. Although such cases attract a great deal of publicity, they are very rare. For a conviction to be successful in terms of gross negligence manslaughter, the prosecution must prove, to the criminal standard, that there was negligence and that the negligence was so gross as to go beyond mere mistake or inattention and such as to warrant a criminal sanction. Again, although such cases do tend to be rare, they are nonetheless important, as they arise not infrequently from systems errors, such as the vinca alkaloid cases, which resulted in the Department of Health issuing a Heath Circular to act as guidance on intrathecal chemotherapy (HSC 2003/010).

Assault

Sexual assault cases often involve allegations of assault upon a female patient by a male doctor, but in any circumstance where an intimate examination is to be performed all doctors should remember the importance of careful and thorough explanation to the patient before the examination and of following the GMC's guidance on chaperones. Although rare, allegations of assault may be made by a patient following a clinical examination or procedure where consent has not been obtained by the treating doctor (see earlier).

Coroners' inquests

Unfortunately, any specialist who deals with very sick patients will experience the death of a patient as an outcome on occasion. The coroner is concerned with unexpected and unnatural deaths. Consequently, it is likely that during their career doctors will have contact with the Coronial Service. The most likely involvement of a doctor is to provide a statement to the coroner (providing a factual account of their attendance on the patient). Hospital trust lawyers are often involved in such cases, and doctors who have drafted a statement may find it useful to discuss its content with the trust's legal team before it is finalized and despatched to the coroner. Similarly, at an inquest, if held, legal representation may be provided by the trust and, unless there is a conflict of interest between the

> the **coroner** is concerned with **unexpected and unnatural deaths**

doctor and the trust, then there is no difficulty in such representation being provided by the hospital as employer. The inquest may be held occasionally with a jury, but most are held with the coroner sitting alone. At the end of the inquest the coroner will arrive at a verdict as to how and by what means a patient died. This may be in the form of a 'traditional' verdict, such as accidental death, misadventure or natural causes, but increasingly coroners are delivering narrative verdicts that set out a detailed account of how a patient died. The coroner does not make findings of civil or criminal liability.

Further reading and resources

British Medical Association & Law Society. *Assessment of Mental Capacity. Guidance for Doctors and Lawyers*, 2nd edn. London: BMJ Books, 2004.

Department of Health. *Maintaining High Professional Standards in the Modern NHS*. London: DH, 2005.
http://www.dh.gov.uk/assetRoot/04/10/33/44/04103344.pdf

Set out under Health Service Circular 2003/012.

Department of Health. *Updated Guidance on the Safe Administration of Intrathecal Chemotherapy*. London: DH, 2005.
http://www.dh.gov.uk/assetRoot/04/06/43/16/04064316.pdf

Set out under Health Service Circular 2003/010.

General Medical Council website: http://www.gmc-uk.org

General Medical Council. *Confidentiality: Protecting and Providing Information*. London: GMC, 2004.
http://www.gmc-uk.org/guidance/current/library/confidentiality.asp

General Medical Council. *Good Medical Practice* London: GMC, 2006.
http://www.gmc-uk.org/guidance/good_medical_practice/index.asp

General Medical Council. *Seeking Patients' Consent: The Ethical Considerations*. London: GMC, 1998.
http://www.gmc-uk.org/guidance/archive/library/consent.asp

General Medical Council. *Tomorrow's Doctors*. London: GMC, 2003 (see paragraph 29).
http://www.gmc-uk.org/education/undergraduate/tomorrows_doctors.asp

Information Commissioner's Office. *Use and Disclosure of Health Data: Guidance on the application of the Data Protection Act 1998*. Wilmslow: ICO, 2002.
http://www.ico.gov.uk/upload/documents/library/data_protection/practical_applicatio n/health_data_-_use_and_disclosure.pdf

the NHS: present and future

'Today, a new relationship is needed between patients and services, and between the health service and the government'
Alan Milburn, Secretary of State for Health (2002)

In July 2000, the NHS Plan was published, which set out radical measures that are far-reaching in their implications and important to comprehend. This followed the mutual recognition by the medical profession, the Government and the NHS of the need to assure and improve the quality of care delivered to patients. The NHS Plan aims, over a period of 10 years, to bring about changes such that the NHS evolves from an organization more geared to its own needs than the needs of the patients to an NHS in which the patients always come first.

the **NHS plan** aims to **put patients first**

The introduction of the NHS Plan, with its focus on decentralization and shifting the balance of power away from Whitehall towards frontline staff, has necessitated changes in the structural organization of healthcare delivery. Although there are regional differences in the way the NHS operates in England and Wales, and in particular in Scotland and Northern Ireland, the broad principles are the same.

Department of Health

The Department of Health (DH) is the Government department responsible for providing NHS organizations, such as hospital trusts and Primary Care Trusts, with the information, guidance and support they need to deliver the Government's policies and meet its standards of patient care. In theory, the DH and the NHS are two separate organizations, and the NHS is not part of the DH. In practice, the DH and the NHS are obviously inextricably interrelated (Figure 7).

Ministers

The DH is run by the Secretary of State, who works with five Ministers for Health. Each of these Ministers for Health has separate responsibilities comprising: social care, long-term care, disability and mental health; performance and quality; public health; emergency care and public involvement; and the NHS.

Departmental leaders

The Departmental leaders comprise:
- board members
- key specialists
- National Clinical Directors
- Directors of Health and Social Care.

The board members are responsible for the day-to-day management of the work of Department and each has individual responsibility for one of the directorates (see below). The most senior board member is the Permanent Secretary of the Department of Health and NHS Chief Executive who reports directly to the Secretary of State for Health.

Key specialists are appointed to provide expert knowledge in the fields of health and social care. They work alongside the Ministers of State for Health and include the Chief Medical Officer, the Chief Social Service Inspector and the Chief Nursing Officer. The Chief Medical Officer is the Government's principal medical advisor and the professional head of all the medical staff in England.

The National Clinical Directors are experts in their field and their roles vary according to their specialty, but include advising on clinical quality and governance.

The four Directors of Health and Social Care form a key part of the new departmental structure. Their work has a territorial focus (London, North, South, Midlands and East of England), but they also have national responsibilities.

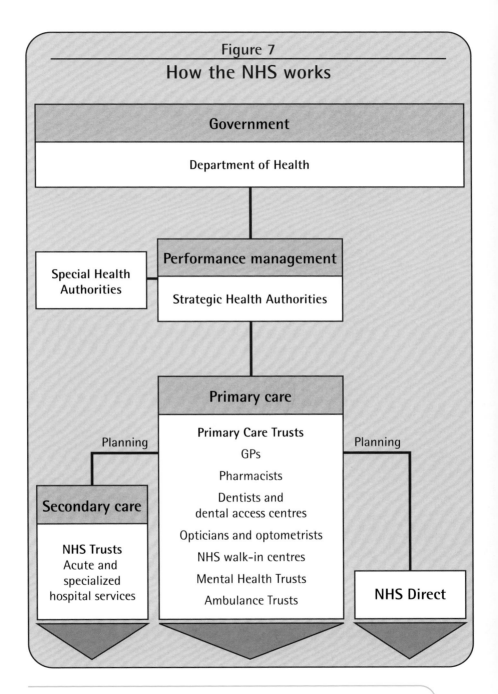

Figure 7

How the NHS works

Government

Department of Health

Performance management

Special Health
Authorities

Strategic Health Authorities

Primary care

Planning

Primary Care Trusts

Planning

GPs

Pharmacists

Secondary care

Dentists and
dental access centres

Opticians and optometrists

NHS Trusts
Acute and
specialized
hospital services

NHS walk-in centres

Mental Health Trusts

NHS Direct

Ambulance Trusts

Directorates

The management board of the DH is made up of a number of directorates, including the Strategy Unit, the Policy Directorate, the Communications Directorate, the Finance Directorate and the Human Resources Directorate.

Executive agencies

The DH works with five executive agencies, which have responsibility for particular areas of healthcare, but are still part of the DH and accountable to it. These are:

- NHS Estates
- NHS Pensions Agency
- Medicines Control Agency
- Medical Devices Agency
- NHS purchasing and supply agency.

Non-departmental public bodies

Aligned with the DH, but separate from it, are various independent executive, advisory and tribunal non-departmental public bodies (NDPBs), which provide specialist advice to the Government about particular areas of work. The eight executive NDPBs include, among others, the English National Board for Nursing, Midwifery and Health Visiting (ENB) and the Commission for Health Improvement. Among the 20 advisory NDPBs are the Committee on the Safety of Medicines and (of more interest to senior hospital doctors!) the Advisory Committee on Clinical Excellence Awards.

Strategic Health Authorities

In April 2002, the 95 health authorities in England ceased to exist and many of their responsibilities were passed to Primary Care Trusts (PCTs, see below). These health authorities have been replaced by much larger Strategic Health Authorities, currently 10, which are responsible for developing strategies and ensuring the quality of the local health service.

Working alongside the Strategic Health Authorities are Special Health Authorities, such as the National Blood Transfusion Service, which provide health services to the whole population, not just to a local community.

Primary Care Trusts

Primary Care Trusts (PCTs) are groups of GP practices and healthcare professionals who work together to provide healthcare for their local area. The approximately 150 PCTs perform many of the duties previously carried out by the regional and district health authorities, and have the funding to purchase secondary care and specialist services in hospitals. This was an area previously handled by the old health authorities and specifically was not given to the new Strategic Health Authorities, which have otherwise taken over most of what the old health authorities used to do. This shift from the regional offices and health authorities to Strategic Health Authorities and PCTs is 'Shifting The Balance of Power', which is how the NHS plan is being implemented. The key point is devolution downwards so that PCTs have the money to purchase secondary and specialist services from hospital trusts whose strategic development is managed by the Strategic Health Authorities, with no direct control over funding issues.

Thus primary care is provided by PCTs through GPs, pharmacists, dentists, optometrists and the NHS walk-in centres. Secondary care is purchased by PCTs and provided by NHS Trusts under the strategic direction of PCTs and the Strategic Health Authorities whose population base encompasses several PCTs.

NHS Direct

NHS Direct offers a free 24-hour telephone advice service to callers.

The NHS Plan

The aim of current government policy is to 'modernize' the NHS, and the basis for this modernization is the NHS Plan, which was published in the year 2000. The NHS Plan is a series of radical reforms to be implemented over a 10-year period with the aim 'to put patients and people at the heart of our health and social services' (Table 26).

Table 26

The NHS Plan

	From	To
A shift in organization and ways of working	• Hierarchical and nationalized • Detailed guidance with many milestones and targets • Focus on institutions	• Devolved local networks • Clear long-term outcomes with latitude about method • Working through networks
A shift in the scale and quality of staff, patient and community involvement	• Small pockets of excellence • Many enthusiasts but not fully embedded • Supported by time-limited 'soft' funding • Many boards still viewing this as peripheral to core business	• Mainstream way of achieving change • Professional and systematic everywhere • Properly resourced through recurring funds • Central to boards' way of working
A shift in management focus	• All management effort driven by delivery of centrally imposed key targets as ends in themselves • Meetings, plans and strategy dominating management time • Risk avoidance because of fear of penalties	• Delivery of targets achieved as the by-product of wider and sustained improvements in service quality • Walking the job with a strong focus on clinical quality • Incentives as a key part of improvement • Penalties seen by all as fair

To drive forward the ideas and improvements outlined in the NHS Plan, the DH has created ten task forces. Six of these task forces will focus on the area that they are intended to improve, namely:

- coronary heart disease
- cancer
- mental health
- older people
- children
- waiting times and access to services.

The remaining four task forces will drive forward the ideas outlined in the NHS Plan, which are:

- the NHS workforce
- quality
- reducing inequalities and promoting public health
- investment in facilities and information technology.

The Modernisation Agency was developed to lead all of these changes. It was chaired by the Secretary of State and included leading figures from healthcare institutions, such as the Royal Colleges, together with representatives from staff and managers within the NHS and patient representatives. The Modernisation Agency had the responsibility to ensure that the commitments laid out in the NHS Plan were translated into reality. After a few years it became clear that such changes were best driven locally and so the Agency, up till then the major driver of these changes, was disbanded and its activities devolved down to trust level.

Quality

The key to the NHS Plan is quality. The Plan describes how quality standards are to be implemented throughout the NHS: first, nationally; secondly, locally; and thirdly, with 'a new organization to address any shortcomings', namely, the Commission for Health Improvement (CHI, subsequently CHAI, now the Healthcare Commission).

At a national level, quality is being addressed in two ways:

- with National Service Frameworks to produce consistency of care for individual clinical categories across the country
- by the reviews of the National Institute for Health and Clinical Excellence (NICE) which determine clinical effectiveness and cost effectiveness of available treatments for disease.

As a result, evidence-based best practice should be available to all patients, wherever they live and whatever their problem. At a local level,

quality is the responsibility of the PCTs, whose aim is to provide healthcare for their local population and who develop service agreements with trusts under the scrutiny and strategic oversight of Strategic Health Authorities. With all of these healthcare providers, quality of patient care at the doctor–patient interface should be ensured by governance.

evidence-based **best practice** should be available to **all patients**

In theory, then, National Service Frameworks for certain clinical conditions ensure that all patients who suffer from these conditions are treated in the same way based on the best available evidence. NICE decides on the basis of the available evidence what the best treatment is and what the most cost-effective approach would be for these and for other clinical conditions. Locally, PCTs purchase these services from hospital trusts under the direction of Strategic Health Authorities, and clinical governance within hospitals ensures that these are enacted locally. Finally, the Healthcare Commission for inspects trusts on a 5-yearly basis to ensure that these principles of quality are put into practice.

Progress so far

In April 2002 the government produced a document, *Delivering the NHS Plan – next steps on investment, next steps on reform*, which, in summary, proposed the model illustrated in Table 27. Specifically, NHS funding was to increase to 9.4% of GDP; waiting times for operations were to drop to 6 months by 2005 and 3 months by 2008; there were to be 15 000 more GPs and consultants and 35 000 more nurses and other healthcare professionals; the hospital payment system was to change to a tariff system called 'payment by results'; patient 'choice' in the booking of outpatient appointments and hospital admissions was to be introduced; diversity (or 'plurality' as it is now called) of service provision from private providers was to be encouraged, particularly for elective surgery; further devolution of the NHS budget to PCTs was to occur; foundation hospitals with increased freedoms were to develop; and there would be

Table 27
The NHS model

	1948 model	New model
Values	● Free at point of need	● Free at point of need
Spending	● Annual lottery	● Planned for 3/5 years
National standards	● None	● National Institute for Health and Clinical Excellence (NICE), National Service Frameworks and single independent healthcare inspectorate/ regulator
Providers	● Monopoly	● Plurality – state, private, voluntary
Staff	● Rigid professional demarcations	● Modernized flexible professions benefiting patients
Patients	● Handed down treatment	● Choice of when and where to get treatment
System	● Top down	● Led by frontline – devolved primary care
Appointments	● Long waits	● Short waits and booked appointments

fundamental changes in job design and work organization leading to new contracts for doctors and for all other healthcare professionals. All of these are happening or have happened.

In June 2005 the NHS Improvement Plan was presented to parliament by the Secretary of State; it went further. Investment in the NHS was to rise from £67 billion in 2004/5 to £90 billion in 2007/8; patients would be admitted for treatment within 18 weeks of referral by their GP and could 'be treated in any facility that meets NHS standards' of their choice and at a time of their choice, with a wider range of services in primary care and near the workplace, the whole process of quality being overseen by the Healthcare Commission.

Choice and the increased capacity to make choice possible are the government's main goals. This increased capacity is to come from 'treatment centres' as well as from traditional private hospitals and other private healthcare providers, supplemented by the (theoretical) stimulus of a tariff system that should (theoretically) encourage trusts, particularly foundation trusts, to make best use of their existing capacity by paying them more than they do now for additional work. Treatment centres, in particular, are highly controversial, but Payment by Results is not without its problems and its full implementation has recently been deferred pending further deliberations. Choice too is struggling because of the lack of technology to implement it, or rather the lack of will to use the technology. Nor do foundation trusts have the freedoms they were initially promised because of the political resistance to their inception and the resistance from the 'centre' which would like to bring them back under central control. The new consultant contract has had its teething problems but is more or less implemented except for clinical academics. Implementation of this is, however, likely to prove to have been simple in comparison with implementation of 'Agenda for Change' for all other healthcare professionals, if only because of the vastly greater number of staff involved.

> **choice** is the government's **main goal**

It is easy, however, to criticize and to point out the problems. It is now clear that most of the NHS Plan is implemented or well on its way, despite a huge dead hand of inertia, if not active opposition. For all we may moan about 'targets', when our nearest and dearest are ill we don't want them to wait 5 minutes in A&E, let alone 4 hours, and doing what is best for our patients, in every respect, is something we would all want to do – if only we had the time and the resources.

The trouble is that for most of us change is coming at a break-neck pace, and that pace seems to be increasing. By the end of 2008 the government expects to have put in place the 18-week wait from the patient's first appointment with the GP to the operation. Currently, maximum waiting times are 13 weeks for outpatients and 6 months for inpatients, so moving to 18 weeks roughly halves the time, effectively doubling the amount of work everybody has to do to achieve the target. At the same time, patient choice has to be allowed for. Hence the 'plurality of provision' that is being pushed, allowing care not only in hospitals and independent treatment centres but also in private hospitals and primary care – that's the way the government hopes the target will be achieved. Incidentally, it is at the end of 2008 too that the year-on-year boost of funding for the NHS will stop.

A range of other new developments is listed in Table 28. The first one to note in particular is the introduction of comprehensive academic medical centres, of which there are to be three in London and one each in Oxford and Cambridge; and six specialist academic medial centres, over half of which are again in London. This is to replace so-called Culyer funding and will allow 'clarity' about how money for research and development is spent so that it can be 'rationalized'.

At the same time as funding for research has been 'rationalized' the Modernising Medical Careers process comes into force, effectively nationalizing training. In 2006, mid-year, the funding for training (the MPET levy) was cut ('rationalized'!).

Table 28

New developments in the NHS

- Best research, best health – academic centres
- Care closer to home
- Centralization – cancer networks
- Diagnostic work
- Day-case targets
- Foundation trusts and the failures
- The independent sector
- Changes in Payment by Results – 'Best Tariff'; pass-through payments
- 18-week target
- General Practitioners with a Special Interest (GPwSI)
- Surgical care practitioners
- New cancer targets for recurrent disease
- European Working Time Directive/Hospital at Night
- Breaking up specialties – disease management
- High-volume–low-risk vs complexity and niche markets, technology
- Modernising Medical Careers

The second point of note is the target to shift work into primary care and the independent sector over the next 2 years in order to make capacity. In 2007, 40% of daycase work is to move. Whether or not it can be moved is another matter, but this is the target.

Finally, and not listed in the table, is the funding squeeze for staff. The GP contract and the consultant contract have proved unexpectedly expensive for the government, with no increase in productivity from the GPs or consultants to show for it. Consultant work plans are being squeezed as this book goes to press, and it is said that the Department of Health workforce group thinks there are 3200 too many consultants, which the Department can't afford to pay (the cost of that number of consultants is about £330 million pounds). So with the consultants and GPs being squeezed by that means, funding for trainees being squeezed by the cut in MPET and with all other health professionals (nurses and paramedical) currently going through the Agenda for Change process it seems likely that there will be a general reduction in either income or medical unemployment; we suspect both.

Supporters will say that all of this will provide increased 'clarity' to allow sensible 'rationalization' of the distribution of resources so as to make the best use of capacity and staff for the best possible service to patients. The sceptic will argue that patients have little or no choice themselves and that it is all designed to weaken the hold of consultants on waiting lists and other facilities; to bring in outsiders to do what has traditionally been the work of secondary care; to provide capacity to do the work outside of traditional secondary care; and to introduce medical unemployment to make the consultant (and other) workforce more compliant.

We will leave it to you to decide.

The future – a change in culture

Changing the organization of the NHS will not, of itself, bring about radical reform. In order for the NHS Plan to be successful, all healthcare staff at every level will need to embrace the change in culture and adopt new attitudes and behaviours.

It remains to be seen how well the NHS plan will function in practice, but it is incumbent on any aspiring hospital doctor who seeks success to know and understand its aims and principles. Central to these reforms is the need for doctors to work together more in teams and less as individuals. 'Multiprofessional' development involving not only doctors, but also other healthcare professionals; flexibility – or 'plurality' – in the provision of healthcare by both individual providers and healthcare organizations; and 'choice' are now the main interests of the DH. Both aspiring and established specialists need to understand these issues and adjust their ideas and their practice accordingly.

Further reading and resources

Department of Health. *Delivering the NHS Plan – next steps on investment, next steps on reform*. 5578. London: DH, 2002.
http://www.dh.gov.uk/assetRoot/04/12/21/93/04122193.pdf

Hawkes N. NHS reorganisation: who's kicking who? *BMJ* 2006;333:645–8.

National Health Service
http://www.nhs.uk

success in medicine: voices of experience

We have invited a selection of 'the great and the good', as well as some of our own friends and colleagues, to give their own recipes for success in medicine. We hope that you will find their stories interesting and their advice useful.

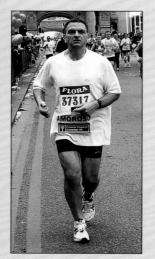

A career in medicine can be all things to all men. However, a new doctor's ambition can quickly become extremely focussed and aimed towards a single goal. The medical student is soon encouraged to choose a path and stick to it up to consultant status and beyond; the hospital trainee can be forgiven for wondering how to change direction once a route is set. But the tremendous thing about medicine is that it offers a rich variety of work, interests and contacts throughout any career. Change at regular intervals ensures continued interest and state-of-the-art practice, whereas endless repetition is undesirable for both practitioner and patients as it leads to complacency and boredom.

In my own case, reinvention has been the key to maintaining my enthusiasm and dedication. As a medical student, I was fortunate to enjoy all disciplines to which I was exposed. Medicine and surgery appealed, but so did pathology and general practice; anaesthesia looked very attractive after my pre-registration year, but I was advised to broaden my training to include accident and emergency. By the end of my house jobs in the mid-1980s, vocational training schemes in general practice were the most competitive posts in the UK. I thought I would enjoy this challenge and began training in one such program, but I continued to enjoy my experience in the field of anaesthesia very much, and I eventually moved into this discipline.

Within anaesthesia, there are so many different areas: pain relief, critical care medicine, maternity, resuscitation or specialist surgical work in theatres. My training covered all these, but I concentrated on research and academic medicine. As a newly appointed consultant in London, I developed my teaching skills and spent a considerable amount of my time teaching – on courses, at the Royal College, in seminar and tutorial work. Later on, I replaced the teaching with training doctors in anaesthesia, a new role for me that replaced the more formal teaching I had previously relished. Later still, I was drawn back to clinical work; I wanted to influence the role of the anaesthetist in the perioperative period. As anaesthetists are physicians with expert skills, it seemed a pity that our skills were only used in 'high-tech' areas of the hospital. I wanted to demonstrate to our patients and colleagues that we could make a difference outside these areas too.

Over two decades, I have been privileged to have experienced all these different areas of anaesthesia and medicine. The opportunities to develop your own skills in an area that suits you are almost limitless. During any one career, professional focus can change from one topic to another, but can often be happily accommodated within a single parent discipline. Anaesthesia has allowed me to develop my people skills with teamwork and talking to patients in the theatre and pain clinic. As a training program director I enjoyed committee work, managing funds and teaching. Currently I have found a new niche in men's health, and I am seeking to develop a new role for the anaesthetist in the perioperative setting. It always seemed to me that the anaesthetist becomes involved in patient care far too late, typically on the day of surgery itself. perhaps a good model of care would be for the anaesthetist to receive a copy of the GP's letter of referral. Teamwork and communication are, after all, paramount for first-class medicine. I believe that the anaesthetist can prepare patients for surgery and help them to improve their fitness, health and nutrition habits so that surgery is less of a risk and their recovery enhanced. We anaesthetists can also assist in counselling and education for the often stressed patients and their family. These objectives make our provision of anaesthesia safer and easier and lead to a great deal of satisfaction for doctor and patient alike.

As obesity and the metabolic syndrome become more widespread in the Western world, the role I propose for anaesthetists will become the greatest task for all doctors, that is, to educate our patients in a healthier lifestyle. The middle-aged men I look after often eat too much, drink too much, smoke too much and regularly work too hard with no exercise; they eat too late in the day and often most unhealthily too. I am a poacher turned gamekeeper here, as I successfully lost 7 stone in weight and then ran the London Marathon in 2002. I am currently setting my sights on the New York Marathon.

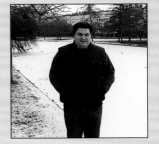

Professor TZ Aziz BSc MBBS MD FRCS FRCS(SN) DMedSci

Department of Neurosurgery, Radcliffe Infirmary, Oxford

Success in medicine is hard to define in the present environment as we struggle to meet ever-changing NHS targets. Nevertheless, here is my story.

I studied physiology as my first degree, initially to understand the nematode neuromuscular junction, but became deeply interested in the control of movement. I saw a film of a thalamotomy in which the surgeon passed an electrode into the motor thalamus of a parkinsonian patient with tremor. When the tip of the electrode was heated, the tremor stopped and normality was restored. That film transformed my life. I became obsessed with the idea that selective destruction of a deep brain target could restore function. I therefore decided to study medicine and make that surgery mine.

Upon qualifying in medicine and then training in neurosurgery I found that such surgery for Parkinson's disease had become obsolete with the introduction of levodopa, a medication that alleviated tremor, rigidity and slowness. However, after a few years patients developed crippling side effects of drug therapy, such as terrible twisting and thrashing of the body. With no understanding of the neural mechanisms of the condition, few advances could be made. Then a primate model of the disease was discovered: giving a pethidine analogue (MPTP) to monkeys rendered them slow, tremulous and stiff, a condition that responded to levodopa. This model revealed that a target deep in the brain, the subthalamic nucleus, was overactive. It seemed possible that destroying this nucleus might improve parkinsonism.

I therefore went to Manchester to research the effects of such surgery in parkinsonian primates. The effects were dramatic, in that all the symptoms were reversed. Soon after publication, it was shown in France that high-frequency stimulation with implanted electrodes had the same effect. This avoided destruction of the nucleus and was more acceptable to clinicians. Today 40 000 people have had such surgery.

Having completed my higher degree I decided that such surgery was my future, but it took fifteen interviews for a senior registrar post before I was appointed. Everywhere I mentioned my ambition I was told the days

Success in medicine: voices of experience

of such procedures were over, until I came to Oxford and was invited to start such a service. So I did, once appointed as consultant after completing the SR period.

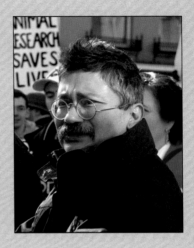

Two years into being a full-time clinician, I felt it was time to return to research. I resigned from 50% of my job and applied for MRC funding to start primate work again. I was interested in the problem that 20% of parkinsonian patients did not respond to medical therapy and conventional surgery did not help them either. With funding from the MRC and with Professor John Stein in physiology, I set out to study the role of the pedunculopontine nucleus in movement. After 10 years of research we were able to show that low-frequency stimulation of the nucleus could reverse slowness of movement in the parkinsonian primate. This work was rapidly taken up clinically and I hope will help many more parkinsonian patients.

Neurosurgery has always fascinated me because of the wonderful opportunities it has given me to study the function of the brain. I am surrounded by a superb team of interested colleagues who share my enthusiasm as we continue studies into movement disorders and pain. I am also grateful to the patients who have taught me so much.

Success, I think, needs belief in oneself and a determination to push one's work through. Now there have been many changes in medical training and the freedom to tailor a career pathway to suit personal interests has been lost; the MMC changes have introduced more rigidity, making it impossible for others to take the pathway that worked for me. If you are interested in pursuing a particular career, it is best to choose much earlier than I had to. Nevertheless, don't rush to finish your training, and enjoy the specialty you have chosen alongside the time to develop outside interests.

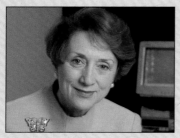

'And the true success is labour', wrote RL Stevenson, a better remark by far, I think, than his more often recalled preceding line 'To travel hopefully is a better thing than to arrive'. There is no easy way to worthwhile achievement, to success. It needs belief, persistence and care to do things well. And to do things better calls for determination and for endurance. But to bring about improvements, to change things – because, as Don Berwick reminds us, without change there is no improvement – means carrying others with you and facing resistance and opposition with conviction, honesty, courage, and stubbornness, and yet still with willingness, however reluctant, to be proved wrong, or even to fail. Those qualities, I suggest, measure Stevenson's idea of success as labour. They are both private and public measures. Without them, is there any real success?

Success for a doctor is favoured by chance. Chance brings the insights offered by each clinical encounter, or through the fresh keen observations of able students, and their disarming questions; or the unexpected or unforeseen experimental result; or the discomforting challenge by people – non-clinicians, with different perspectives, different responsibilities and other priorities.

For the hospital doctor, success neither can be nor should be a solitary experience. Ours is a corporate business, though I prefer the term 'collegiate', with its sense of a wide-reaching shared enterprise securely anchored by a professionalism whose sustenance and improvement are measures of success that really matter.

Professor John Blandy CBE FRCS

Department of Urology, Royal London Hospital

One measures success by the size of his Rolls-Royce; another by the number of letters after his name. Let me dodge the issue and discuss happiness.

To begin with, you need luck: luck in health, luck in the person you marry, luck in your children. If you are honest, little of this is down to your choice or your cleverness: luck again.

Next to luck comes interest. Odd pathology is always turning up just when least expected; there is always some exciting new technical development. In my surgical lifetime I suppose the first big event was learning transurethral resection in Chicago and trying to teach it to my younger colleagues in London. Later came the challenges of staghorn calculi, urethral strictures and renal transplantation, followed by the excitement of the schemes to get each transplant matched for LHA. These were days when I found myself working in collaboration with real scientists such as Hilliard Festenstein and Tim Oliver, who dazzled me with their flights of imagination, even if I seldom fully understood them.

Interest is not enough, either. You need to kindle enthusiasm in others. You must write up the bees in your bonnet. If you do a lot of one particular operation, you owe it to your patients and your team to keep the score and report it. Today some of this is compulsory under audit, but it should be done out of interest, for its own sake.

Much of the pleasure in my life as a working surgeon came from the enjoyment of the people with whom I worked: above all my patients, but also everyone else – the nursing staff in outpatients and the theatre; my colleagues in anaesthesia, radiology and pathology. Seldom does one have much choice in whom one works with, so if you find them fun you are lucky. I certainly was.

Rodney Burnham MA MD FRCP

Registrar, Royal College of Physicians;
Consultant Physician, Gastroenterologist and Honorary Senior Lecturer,
Barking, Havering & Redbridge NHS Trust; Barts and the London School of Medicine

As a young doctor, I worked in Africa for a year at a mission hospital. I intended to contribute, but in fact I gained more than I ever gave. The hospital superintendent was a modest, dedicated and gifted Christian man, described by a UK professor of surgery as a 'surgical genius'. He had never published a paper, written a book or achieved national recognition. Without ambition beyond the welfare of his patients, he was nevertheless a very successful hospital doctor and great leader. He believed, as I do, that the gifts and abilities that enable success were given to us and that we have a responsibility to use them well. The successful apostle Paul said:

> *For what makes you different from anyone else? What do you have that you did not receive? And if you did receive it, why do you boast as if you did not?* (Letter to the Church at Corinth)

At the start of my consultant post, I set myself three objectives: to provide the best possible service to my patients; to teach doctors in training working with me; and to undertake research and audit. It was very satisfying to discover 5 years later that I had achieved much of what I had set out to do, but circumstances change and produce new challenges. Success is as much about adapting to these as it is about achieving one's original objectives.

A management consultant emphasizes that successful leaders have a 'stop doing' list. A successful consultant will avoid seeking success solely for money, possessions, power or position and will not take any action or decision that lowers ethical standards. A colleague once asked me during

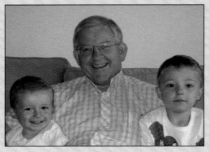

a local medico-political difficulty: 'Why can't you say yes and mean no?' But honesty and integrity are essential for success.

Finally, one must take care not to neglect responsibilities at home. One of the best indicators of success is a good family life. My wife, three children and two grandsons bring me great contentment.

Success in medicine: voices of experience

Linda Cardozo MD FRCOG

Professor of Urogynaecology, King's College Hospital, London

Success in medicine – as in any other career – can be judged in many different ways, and I am not sure that I would consider myself to be successful. Some think of me as intolerant and undiplomatic with a dreadful bedside manner. I don't really like hospitals or the way in which the NHS is currently being managed, nor do I approve of the new system of training doctors. In addition, I can't cope with ill health in myself, family or friends; so I am not really the ideal doctor. However, I am enthusiastically dedicated to my career in medicine and have developed my own ten commandments.

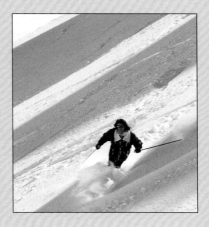

1. You really can have your cake and eat it. Don't believe anyone who says you cannot have a successful career in clinical medicine with a good reputation in your hospital, an international research profile, a busy private practice and a happy family life – it is possible, you just have to engineer it. Work hard, play hard; it is not worth doing the former without the latter.

2. Appropriate time management is essential. Don't waste time. I was influenced by Golda Meir's autobiography *My Life* in which she emphasized the importance of striving to do a little more each day than she had managed during the previous one. Punctuality at work is essential: not only does it set a good example and stop the trainees from turning up late, but it ensures that the operating lists don't overrun, thus pleasing the anaesthetist and theatre staff. However, social activities can often be delayed; no one really minds or even notices when you go round to a friend's half an hour or an hour late, giving you time to get your slides ready for tomorrow's lecture or mark the last few exam papers before you go.

3. Delegate – it is not possible to do everything yourself, nor is it

---

Succeeding as a hospital doctor

desirable. The people you train usually do things your way, only better, so let them.

4. Think to whom it matters most. Whenever you have a dispute at work or at home, try to be one who gives in unless you are absolutely certain that winning is essential to you. It is not worth upsetting people for something that is of minor importance.

5. Don't 'criticize' your colleagues. You never know when you'll need their help. Try to support them when they are in dispute with others and don't be frightened to ask for their help when you need it. Protect your boss – everyone is hungry for something and you are bound to need him or her for a reference, surgical training or teaching in the future.

6. Develop a way of saying 'no' without causing offence. It is flattering to be asked and tempting to accept all invitations to lecture, operate abroad, examine and write, but it is impossible to do it all. Try to judge which events it would be possible to miss and offer a member of your team instead.

7. Give others the opportunity to do things they wouldn't have otherwise been able to do. This applies to patients, colleagues, family and friends. Don't do it for them, but give them the facilities, advice, time and financial aid to do it for themselves. It is much more rewarding for you and for them.

8. Make use of all the support services you can. It is much quicker to earn the money to pay a secretary to do the typing, a cleaner to do the housework and a gardener to mow the lawn than it is to do it yourself. If at all possible, marry an understanding spouse and teach your family to appreciate that medicine isn't just a job, it's a way of life.

9. It's not enough to fulfil your contract, you have to show commitment by starting early, staying late and taking on extra tasks, including teaching, research and committee work.

10. Enjoy life – if you are not happy most of the time, then change tack. Life is too short to spend time being miserable!

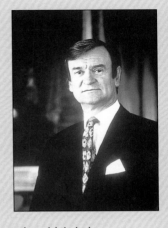

It helps to succeed in medicine if you remember that it is not only a science, but an art too. I interned in the USA, alongside colleagues better technically trained than me. However, they placed much less emphasis on communication with patients than me. I quickly saw how important it is to be not only able, but also willing to communicate with patients – in terms of improved patient compliance, avoiding confrontations with patients or relatives, fostering a more realistic attitude to what medicine can and cannot do – for example, being able to tell a patient that there is nothing more that can be done while still maintaining a fruitful doctor–patient relationship.

Many doctors, indeed most of us, work in situations in which being able to accept the limits of what they can do is absolutely essential to their survival as doctors. A number of very wise physicians have taught me that medicine's therapeutic enthusiasm, essential for the most part, has its own drawbacks. Doctors can have difficulty accepting their limits, and end up making such needless and pointless effort.

Finally, there is the issue of pacing yourself. Read William Osler's *A Way of Life* and ponder his regret that many a young medical life has been wrecked by too fast a starting pace, a hustle, bustle and tension, 'the human machine driven day and night'. Avoid what William James has called 'those absurd feelings of hurry and having no time', and always leave room for the important things in your own personal life – your loves, family and friends. That way you can, even in the most awesomely demanding situations, call each day your own and be not just a good doctor but perhaps even a great one.

'Medicine is a noble profession.' So replied a prospective applicant to medical school years ago when I asked why he wanted to be a doctor. Throughout my career in medicine, I haven't seen too much evidence of nobility, but I have found that an undue obsession with status or too great a fondness for the trappings of high professional life can be dangerous traits. A doctor who is an autocratic leader, who regularly has disputes with colleagues or who is unable to see the world through the eyes of the ordinary patient is likely to be associated with dysfunctional clinical teams, risking poor outcomes for patients.

After training in surgery, I moved into epidemiology and public health, initially in an academic role and later as director of public health for one of the NHS regions. For 6 years, I combined this role with that of regional director (effectively chief executive). Appointment as the Government's Chief Medical Officer means that I have now worked in all six sectors that make up British healthcare – hospital medicine, primary care, public health, academic medicine, management and the Government service.

I have learned that while the technical tasks of medicine are important, it is at the level of the team, the service and the organization that good healthcare is generated. Achieving results through people and managing change is a universally difficult task and one that few are skilled in, trained or prepared for. Many of tomorrow's doctors will be in leadership roles. They will need to create the culture in which excellence in clinical decision-making can flourish.

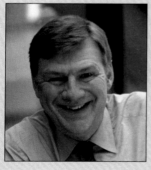

Many of the qualities needed are well captured in the expression 'the reflective practitioner'. Someone who is willing to learn and change, someone who is willing to listen, someone who seeks feedback on their performance and someone who is willing to reassess a misunderstanding is more likely to take the right decision in a complex clinical situation or when the future of a service is being debated. Such a person is more likely, too, to gain the respect of peers and colleagues as a clinical leader.

Success in medicine: voices of experience

Harold Ellis CBE DM MCh FRCS

Emeritus Professor of Surgery, University of London

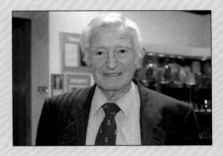

I came from a completely non-medical family, but I found biology to be an especially interesting subject in my sixth form at school. My biology master, who I particularly admired, told me that in those days (1940), as a keen biologist, I could either become a science master like him or become a doctor. Without a moment's hesitation I chose the latter, and I have never regretted it.

In my opinion, being a doctor – and especially being a surgeon – is to be part of the greatest of the professions. What other vocation allows you to spend your working life helping people who are in pain, or disfigured, or crippled, return to a normal or at least a reasonable life? In most jobs you end your working day by estimating how much you have earned; as a doctor, you measure how many people you have succoured.

What attributes do you need to be a good doctor?

- First, you certainly have to be intelligent. There is a mass of material you need to learn; more than learn, that you have to understand and appreciate as a doctor. If you are not bright enough, this learning process will prove to be a terrible struggle and you will just not qualify. I am convinced that it is right and proper that medical schools insist on high academic grades as an essential entry requirement.

- Second, you need to be a hard worker. There is an enormous amount that you need to assimilate in your training, both before and even more after qualification, and your training will go on throughout your career. If you want an easy ride, then do not choose medicine.

- Third, and the most important of the three, you need to have a real love of your fellow human beings and a real desire to help them, whether they be rich or poor, pleasant or unpleasant, clean and tidy or dirty and smelly.

What about my own specialty of surgery? Do you need to be of extraordinary natural dexterity? Well, certainly you can never be taught to operate if you are all fingers and thumbs, but trainees self-select. Young graduates do not choose this specialty if they are not adequately competent with their hands to be trained to become effective operators.

The tyro surgeon does need to face a life of hard physical and mental work. Four or five hours removing a difficult stuck tumour in a hot operating theatre does require a lot of physical and mental concentration.

So how does the student learn to become a 'good doctor'? Studying the textbook is important, but is entirely overshadowed by a lifetime of studying your patients. I can do no better than to give you my favourite quotation, which I am always passing on to my students, and which is from that great teacher, Sir William Osler:

> To study the phenomena of disease without books is to sail on uncharted seas, while to study books without patients is not to go to sea at all.

I began to keep records of my patients on cards as a student, and continued to do so until I retired from clinical work and returned to teaching students anatomy, and I beseech them to do the same.

My final piece of advice is this: choose your spouse with the very greatest care. My own dear wife brought up the children, ran the home while I was long hours in the hospital or away abroad, and encouraged me and comforted me during the trials and disappointments that accompany any career. Without her, I would have been as nothing.

Michael Farthing

Principal and Professor of Medicine, St George's, University of London

When I greet our fresher medical students during their first week, I tell them that 'I am a man of few words', and that they only have to remember six words: 'Work hard, have fun, be good'. At their graduation ceremony I tell them (and their long-suffering parents) that there are two more... 'Get paid!'

This mantra is, I believe, still relevant to the successful practice of hospital medicine. Although there are increasing concerns about 'life-work balance', I still believe in the perhaps old-fashioned adage that 'the more you put in, the more you get out'.

Make sure you are doing something you really want to do and that you have a plan to get to where you want to be – your vision and mission. Choose your future colleagues carefully. Many, perhaps most, consultants remain in the same post for most of their working life. A warm, supportive relationship with other close colleagues is probably the next most important factor for maintaining your sanity and achieving personal success.

Despite the reduction in working hours, hospital practice will remain a challenging and demanding profession. If it is not working out, have the courage to change. The skills to manage change have never been more important. Be prepared to reinvent yourself every 10 years. It will enrich both your professional and personal life.

After the first 10 years of specialist practice you will be a highly skilled clinician and be able to function for much of the time on 'autopilot'. During the next phase of your career, routine clinical practice may lose some of its appeal. You will, however, continue to learn from your patients, who in my experience often become more interesting than the diseases from which they suffer! A parallel interest in research and/or education and training will enhance your professional development when you perhaps feel overwhelmed by the cyclothymia of the NHS.

Succeeding as a hospital doctor

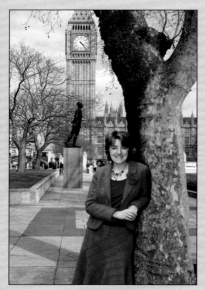

There is a Japanese saying, 'Success is fall down seven times, get up eight times'. My career path has not been straightforward, and indeed the speciality of palliative medicine did not exist when I first became involved full time in caring for the terminally ill. But if you are motivated in your work, believe in what you are doing and ensure that you approach the subject with an open mind and constantly learn, then you can develop as a doctor and contribute to the society around you. There are no shortcuts or alternatives to hard work. Medicine is a constantly changing and expanding field, throwing up research questions faster than they can be answered. In our rapidly changing society those who are ill can feel vulnerable, frightened and undervalued as people. In providing care it is always worth thinking how you yourself would like to be cared for and remembering that attention to detail is crucial in ensuring that the patient as a person, as well as the patient's disease, is treated appropriately.

And the day that you become hardened to the plight of patients is the day to retire.

Sir JA Muir Gray CBE MD FRCP(Glas & Lond)

Programmes Director, National Screening Committee;
Director, National Library for Health

I have found the following proverbs and epigrams particularly apt with regard to my own career, remembering the most useful definition of a 'career' is that it is the name given to all those crazy decisions one has made in the past 20 years.

- Montgomery said, 'There is only one rule in war – never invade Russia'. Always identify and avoid impossible tasks.
- Having decided that you are going to have a crack at something, remember the motto of the Chindits – the boldest course is the safest.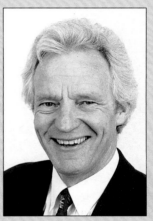
- Success in a project is often the result of chance, failure the result of bad planning and execution; failures are more important than successes for learning.
- Never put your faith in organizations, only in people.
- Fortunate is the doctor whose main source of stress is his patients; most doctors I know have more stress caused by colleagues.
- It is easier to seek forgiveness than permission.

As I write this column, a 'leak' of the of the draft NHS pay and workforce strategy (2007) claims 'an excess supply of 3200 consultants which we cannot afford to employ'. My consultant friends tell me that there has been a complete freeze of recruitment in many hospitals and that no-one dare blow the whistle about the knock-on effects this is having on patient care for fear of falling foul of 'natural wastage'.

Meanwhile, profiteering overseas health corporations – having saturated the market in their own countries – are using the NHS as their gateway into Europe. As the government waves them in with guaranteed contracts, paid above tariff whether they do the work or not, they're busy cherry-picking the easy stuff and leaving district general hospitals to mop up anyone unfortunate enough to be too sick to turn a profit.

Hospitals, saddled with the obligation to treat everyone, just can't compete; particularly those also saddled with a £100-million-a-year PFI debt before they even open their doors. 'Healthcare outside hospitals' aims to strip down district general hospitals as much as possible, with outpatients fobbed off onto GPs (with or without special interests). And casualty departments and maternity units are being culled under a process of 'reconfiguration' without any obvious evidence base.

In a year when record investment in the NHS ended with record debt, the focus is entirely on balancing the books. Just about anything in the NHS that can be done cheaper by those with fewer qualifications is being done, never mind the quality. For the first time, doctors have joined the real world of job insecurity. Some can't get jobs, others can't hold onto the ones they have. *Succeeding as a Hospital Doctor* sounds more like irony than reality.

The government has deliberately destabilized hospital doctors, allowing unfair competition from private treatment centres with no published outcome data, and the suspicion is that they want you all to retreat into chambers and join the frantic scramble for work. We still have the trust of the public, but I'm not sure enough of us will unite en masse to defend the principles of the NHS. In my own specialty, general practice, a two-tier labour market has developed, with partners taking large profits and sweatshop assistants doing the work and earning less than £40 an hour. The same discontent will fester for sub-consultant grades, but with so few jobs around doctors are accepting poor pay and training.

In such a system, successful doctors are likely to be those with a strong entrepreneurial spirit who diversify and compete. In many areas, GPs have clumped together to form commissioning consortia to take on the might of the multinationals. Consultants too are setting up limited companies with slick advertising and published results. Show you're better than the competition and patients will come to you. Sit back and sulk, and they won't.

I diversified back in 1990, first as a comedian, then as a journalist, lecturer, writer and broadcaster. For sixteen years, I've earned more analysing and satirizing the NHS than I have working in it. I still do a few sessions a week to keep in touch, but it's the inability of politicians to sort out the NHS that keeps me in business. Our obsession with health shows no signs of waning, and there's still a huge market out there for doctors who can talk and write about what's happening. And the more successful you are, the more you can tell it like it is, safe in the knowledge that you've got a living outside the NHS. It's a risk to start with, but if you pull it off it's both lucrative and liberating.

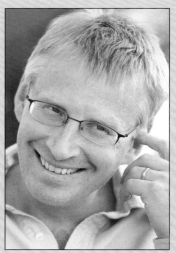

I believe the most important single attribute that leads to success, whether in medicine or in other fields, is enthusiasm. Fortunately, although enthusiasm is not something that you are born with, it can be acquired. Like a fire, enthusiasm must be sparked initially. Thereafter, it should be fuelled; finally, it can be fanned into flames that cannot be extinguished.

Just so in medicine: a great teacher shares enthusiasm for his subject with his students. Whether it be cardiac surgery or cataracts, volvulus or varicose veins, the intense interest of the individual teacher is conveyed. In my case, it was kidney disease that first stirred enthusiasm: young people dying of uraemia while a dialysis machine lay in the next room, only used for acute reversible renal failure. The idea of organ transplantation was not new, but the dream of new organs to replace those that had failed inspired an enormous international effort that saw kidney transplantation become a reality.

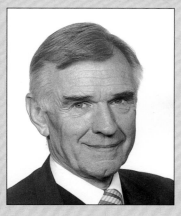

Enthusiasm is catching. A teacher with a needle-sharp mind, absolute clarity of vision and communication skills can shed light where before there were obscurity and darkness. We have all seen the results – a group of students fired into activity, competing to produce the best dissertation, and falling over each other to get onto the ward round or into the operating theatre, questions waiting to be answered. And life choices to be made: will it be medicine for the thoughtful, surgery for the practical or pathology for the reflective? So long as there is enthusiasm, success is sure to follow.

Professor Janet Husband OBE FMedSci

Department of Radiology, Royal Marsden Foundation NHS Trust, London

Within medicine success can be measured in various different ways, and there are of course many unsung heroes who should be ranked amongst the most successful. So what is my definition of success? I believe it is simply the ability to make a difference, whether it be a difference to individual patients, a difference to our specialties or a difference to the profession as a whole. Some of us are privileged to be in a position to influence the development and advancement of our specialties and our profession, but being in such a position carries heavy responsibilities both to patients and to the profession. Nevertheless, such responsibilities are frequently balanced by a fruitful and rewarding career.

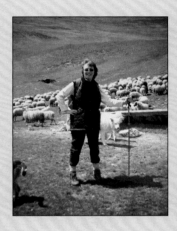

So what then is the secret of such a successful career? Well, in my view there are four key ingredients.

First and foremost, it is vitally important that work is fun and that you are filled with energy, excitement and enthusiasm to achieve the highest possible standards in all you that you do. You should take every opportunity that comes your way in building your career. You won't get a second chance!

Secondly, you must be able to make a contribution and to help others to achieve their own objectives. At the end of each day it is good to reflect on what you have achieved and to define goals for the next. In this way you will always be travelling forward and will aspire to new goals, some of which you may have thought were previously beyond your reach.

Thirdly, you should continually learn and grow through your everyday experiences throughout your career. Always be ready to recognize the talents of others and learn from their expertise and experience.

Finally, you do need a little bit of luck along the way!

If you adhere to these principles and have a little bit of luck, I believe you will be successful.

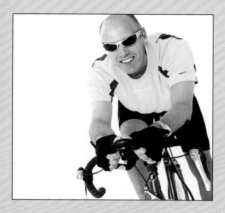

For an academic, career success requires the juggling of the, sometimes contradictory, requirements imposed by the NHS and the university. This effectively gives multiple domains by which career success or failure can be judged – personal goals (both academic and clinical); personal non-career goals; peer and patient assessment of clinical success and peer assessment of academic success. All areas require constant attention, and sometimes effort in one area, such as family and home life, will subtract from potential for delivery in another area, such as the successful writing of another key grant application. This makes a successful career rather like spinning plates – you have to give enough attention to each domain to keep them all going, but cannot attend to all at the same time. Others may take a different view and consider a successful career to involve spinning one very large plate!

My first thoughts on defining success were to think back to who had impressed me as a student and junior doctor. The first defining feature was that all team members were listened to and valued; strong leadership does not require a dictatorship. The second feature was that successful teams were those where the patient was the focus of the team effort, coupled with a relentless attention to detail: making sure the i's were dotted and the t's crossed. Inevitably, if this is done, everything else will follow. When patients are poorly managed it is usually, in my opinion, because the basics have not been done correctly, not because someone failed to spot an obscure sign from a rare illness. In particular, not taking an accurate history often underlies subsequent poor decision-making. A key take-home message from sitting the ritualistic undergraduate and postgraduate clinical exams in the 1980s was that if you didn't know the diagnosis by the time you got your stethoscope out you were probably sunk, and I think this true of medicine in general, not just examinations.

In conclusion, I think the key to a successful career is to try and maximize outcomes in the different domains that make up a professional life. This will mean much hard work and some compromise between areas; too much emphasis on success in one area at the expense of the others will not in the long run lead to a successful, satisfying career.

Parveen J Kumar CBE BSc MD FRCP FRCP(E)

President of the British Medical Association, 2006–07;
Professor of Clinical Medical Education, Barts and the London, Queen Mary School
of Medicine; Consultant Gastroenterologist, Barts and the London NHS Trust
and Homerton Hospital NHS Foundation Trust

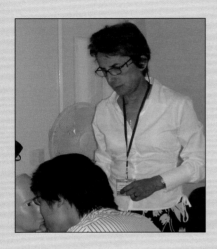

I have been extremely fortunate in having a career that I enjoy, and I look forward to going into work every morning. I had always wanted to do medicine as it combined the two things that I wanted in a fulfilling career: science and caring for people. We are fortunate as doctors to be able to do both, but there is no denying that it is very hard work. Medicine can be so all-embracing that if you are not careful it can take over the whole of your life. Rewards are few – but when they come, can sustain you for a long time. The best is a simple 'thank you' from a patient who has recovered from an illness.

I didn't actually plan my career but just took up the opportunities that I thought I would enjoy as they came my way. So, as I grew up (!) my career moved (with a constant background of clinical work) to research, writing a textbook, teaching and education. I had always been dissatisfied with the ghastly, turgid medical texts that I had to learn from when I was a student. This led me, with my co-editor, to develop a new type of textbook with illustrations, figures and algorithms along with colour; it had to be fun to learn from. Thus Kumar and Clark's *Clinical Medicine* came into being, and since then has been a wonderful way for me to keep up-to-date! I also love teaching, as I learn so much from the students and young doctors – and they certainly can be challenging. Of course, I also have a lot of committee work – time-consuming, but worth it if you can make a difference.

To balance all the above, it is imperative that you have a life outside medicine. Mine has been my family, but it has not always been easy to combine medicine with bringing up a family. My husband was a great support, particularly at a time when there were few women in medicine.

Choose your spouse well! Then you need other interests; mine include skiing (particularly with the family), walking and opera.

So, my tips for a good career in medicine are:

- always be prepared to say you don't know and ask for help (this can be difficult sometimes, but is nevertheless a must)
- never be arrogant (it usually means you are ignorant!) or pompous
- remember the patient is the most important person
- treat everyone as you would like to be treated yourself.
- and, above all, have FUN!

Professor Gordon McVie MD FRCP

Clinical Research Director, European Institute of Oncology, Milan

I suppose I became a consultant at 31 because I was in a novel specialty and I was around at the right time. Anti-cancer drugs were just being developed in the early 1970s. I was in an excellent clinical pharmacology and haematology unit and was lucky enough to be given training in the USA, thanks to the late Gordon Hamilton-Fairley, the first Professor of Medical Oncology in the UK. He was blown up, tragically, as most people

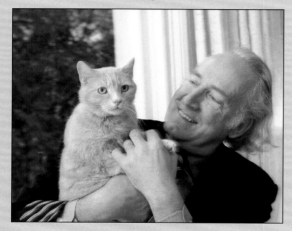

will remember, by mistake by an IRA bomb. So how did I get to the consultant job at an early age? An outstanding professor, who gave me a rope long enough to hang myself, and a determination, particularly after Hamilton-Fairley's death, to pick up the reins and fill the gap – I think if you ask any number of medical oncologists why they are doing what they are doing, they will also attribute the motivation to Hamilton-Fairley. But more fundamentally, I had started off life with genetically endowed curiosity. This was hammered out of me at school while I swotted for exams to escape from school and I humdrummed my way through university, only finding the library when invited to do an honours degree in pathology. I recovered my curiosity within the library and it has not been dampened since!

Success in medicine: voices of experience

Anthony W Nathan MD FRCP FACC FESC FHRS

Consultant Cardiologist, St Bartholomew's Hospital, London

Medical success can be judged in at least two ways:

- Personal happiness and contentment (how it feels from the inside)
- Esteem from one's patients and peers (how it looks from the outside).

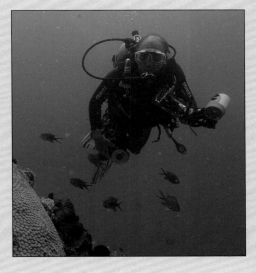

I believe that true success (fulfilment) combines the two, but what feels like success to one doctor may be different for another. Some may want a 'simple' life concentrating on the provision of good clinical care, whilst others may want a more complex existence and seek political position, international reputation, financial gain and so on. Some create adequate time for family and personal life while others may sacrifice this for 'professional success'. One isn't necessarily better than the other – fortunately we all aspire to different types of career.

I have always yearned for variety and have sought a career which would allow me to change the focus of my work over the years. I never wanted a quiet life, and wanted to be a specialist from the day I first worked in a hospital. My career has included the development, delivery and teaching of new techniques in interventional electrophysiology, active involvement in national and international societies and more recently running the Barts and The London Heart Centre.

To achieve what I perceive as success, I recommend the following 10-point plan:

1. Be honest with yourself as to the type of life you want, how hard you really want to work and how important your home life is to your overall happiness.
2. Know what your strengths and weaknesses are.

3. Have a basic career plan, but don't be afraid to deviate from it and do take any significant opportunities that present themselves.
4. Try to anticipate where medicine is going, and think about the opportunities that are likely to exist by the time that you are trained.
5. Make sure you have the best teachers available at *all* stages of your life.
6. Make yourself indispensable, especially if an in-house opportunity might arise.
7. Ask for advice from those you trust, and act on it. Never be afraid to discuss anything (especially clinical problems) at any stage.
8. Constantly put yourself in the position of others, whether patients, colleagues, managers or politicians. Do to others what you would like done to yourself!
9. Seek support, back-up and tolerance from your family and friends.
10. Take time to indulge yourself and look after your own well-being. Always ensure that life is fun and enjoyable.

Academic medicine contains wonderful opportunities, combining research, teaching and clinical practice. The mix will vary over your career, and I think it is really important to be open to the opportunities that will present themselves to you; if an opening comes up in an area that excites you, then go for it hard. I originally thought I might go into full-time neuroscience research when I was an undergraduate, but decided to complete

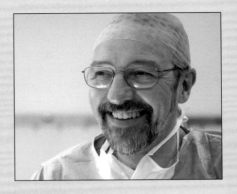

my clinical training. Somewhat to my surprise, I really enjoyed surgery and decided that academic urological surgery was for me, though only after I had done a fair bit of general surgery and urology. The thing that made a difference was coming across people who really enjoyed what they did. Academic surgery, which combines clinical practice, the development and honing of practical skills, and establishing research projects, requires luck and the recognition and willingness to seize opportunities that come up; and it requires hard work, commitment and enthusiasm.

Medicine is a team game, and it requires excellent communication skills, which include highly developed listening skills – targeted at colleagues as well as patients!

A real danger for British medicine is that we could lose confidence in what we do and forget our role in maintaining professionalism and clinical leadership within healthcare. The politicians should of course set the broad agenda, but in recent years there has been too much micromanagement, which has been extremely damaging. Nevertheless, the future for academic medicine and academic surgery is really bright, in my view; the young people we are recruiting are first class.

My experience within the NHS is that the system is somewhat complex and can stifle initiative and excellence, so you need to circumvent many of these obstacles and sometimes ignore the rules. Pick a subject you enjoy and make it your own!

Doctors who practise, as opposed to those who preach, can find themselves out of tune with the managerial ethos that dominates our culture. One reason, I suspect, is that it harps so much on success, as if that were the ultimate human achievement. Yet doctors practise a craft in which the ultimate 'outcome' is a patient's death. And much of the art of medicine – well, the sort of medicine I want practised on me – is concerned with trying to help people survive the short spell they have on this earth in some sort of harmony with the world around them.

George Orwell suggested that, seen from within, every life is a succession of failures. Experience has taught me that failure doesn't matter. A lesson I learned in clinical medicine – and now apply to less worthy activities – is that life can still be rewarding if you strive for perfection while knowing you're unlikely to achieve it. Maturity dawns when failure becomes a worthy objective. You can fail only if you try to do something; the surest route to success is doing nothing.

I hope Valhalla has a special hall for those whom success-chasers call 'losers': a European navigator, maybe, who got to America ten years before

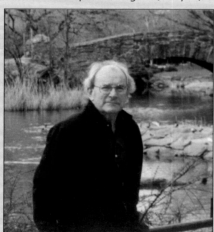

Columbus but liked it so much he didn't bother to come home to boast of his success. Valhalla would need a much grander hall for those who know they are successful: the 17th-century intellectuals, for instance, who said of Galileo, 'He's a decent enough chap but he's got this fixation about Copernicus. Insists the earth moves round the sun when he just needs to stick his head out the window to see he's wrong.'

Professor Sir Michael Rawlins BSc MD FRCP FFPM FMedSci
Chairman, National Institute for Health and Clinical Excellence

I am not entirely sure what success is about; I am not at all sure that I have been a successful hospital doctor. Nevertheless, if professional success is about anything, it is about fulfilment. It is not about honours, titles and merit awards which are as much concerned with luck as anything else, but about deriving the greatest satisfaction from giving all patients (especially the nasty ones) the highest attainable standards of clinical care.

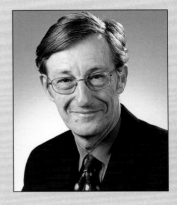

There are a number of essential ingredients to success, learned painfully over a long period of time, to which I aspire.

- Humility. Never be too proud to ask colleagues for help or advice.
- Hard work. Nothing useful is achieved without effort. Success will not come from keeping 'office hours'. Don't get too upset if you are described as a 'workaholic'.
- Humanism. One day you, too, will be a patient, so treat all patients (even the unpleasant ones) as you would wish to be treated yourself.
- Humour. Interject, at appropriate times, a little levity.
- Honesty. When you make a mistake (as we all do), at least admit it – if only to yourself. But to really succeed, you must also be prepared to say you are sorry!
- Honour. Respect and cherish those who work with and for you. Never abuse your position, or their trust, by bullying or humiliating them.
- Hours. Make sure you spend some time away from work with your family and friends. And give yourself 'thinking time' as you mow the lawn, paint the kitchen, clean the car or drive to work. It is in those situations that you will be at your most creative.

Charles Rodeck BSc MBBS DSc(Med)
FRCOG FRCPath FMedSci

Professor of Obstetrics and Gynaecology, University College London;
Director of Fetal Medicine Unit, University College Hospital

We are all shaped by three interacting forces: our genes, our placenta, which determines our prenatal environment, and our parents, who provide our postnatal environment. Of these, the placenta is the most important, because some compensation can usually be made for deficiencies in the other two, but a bad placenta leads to death, to irreversible abnormalities of growth, development or intellectual function, or to disease in later life. 'He would say that – he's an obstetrician', I hear you say, but it's true!

We can exercise no choice over these three basics, but assuming that they are satisfactory, how does one succeed as a hospital doctor? To define success would take too long, so I will get to the point by saying that the most important quality is *ambition*. Not ambition for the false idols of power or wealth, but ambition to excel at being a clinician. This requires a passionate desire to get it right for the patient and to avoid making mistakes and causing harm; to establish a partnership with patients based on honesty, humility and trust; to ensure that patients feel better after seeing you than before, even if you have to tell them of a catastrophe, such as their fetus having a severe abnormality. These are skills that can only be learned by apprenticeship, sitting in on consultations rather than in lectures.

If you are considering clinical academia, you need to be good at several other things: research, teaching, administration, leadership. You must value knowledge but be sceptical, never be bored or waste time, or need more than 5 hours' sleep! You must be prepared to be different in order to make a difference; to have original research questions or to do something that others have not done before. At the start of my career, for example, fetal medicine did not exist. It is now a major subspecialty and I am proud to have contributed towards that change.

Ambition can be dangerous! It must be tempered by another cardinal quality, *judgement*, which is allied to discrimination and a sense of proportion. You need these to ensure you make the right decisions in selecting jobs, career path and the specialty that you enjoy and in which you will make your mark. For me, obstetrics was simply the most exciting subject; here, decision-making and timing are paramount, with an element of risk and danger usually culminating (thankfully) in a happy outcome. At a more senior level, decisions have wider repercussions than your own career.

Guiding principles are:

- aim to appoint people more able than yourself;
- help them up, don't keep them down;
- try to leave your department in better shape than when you arrived.

It is a source of great satisfaction to me that twelve of my former trainees and co-workers have chairs in this country or abroad.

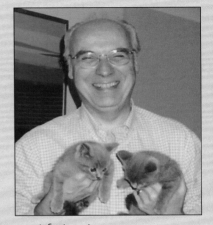

Judgement is also needed in balancing work with family and outside interests. However, beware of the European Working Time Directive, which appears to be affecting this to the detriment of work.

Last but not least, your choice of partner is crucial. Stability, support, understanding, tolerance (and laughter) at home are essential and not always easy to give. In that I have been most fortunate.

Marcus Setchell CVO FRCS FRCOG

Consultant Obstetrician and Gynaecologist, Whittington Hospital,
and Honorary Consultant, St. Bartholomew's and Homerton Hospitals

Despite our current preoccupation with targets, outcome measures, audit and standardization of training and clinical care, there remain many criteria by which success may be measured or perceived. The diversity of medicine is one of the reasons why it is still such an attractive career, allowing individuals to make their contribution to society in many different ways.

Some young doctors set their goals at an early stage of their training, whilst others need to taste a variety of medical and environmental experiences before they find their niche. Early target setting may be admirable, but retaining openness and flexibility can be equally valuable. Opportunities sometimes present themselves unexpectedly. Be prepared to stretch or test yourself, for example by applying for a job that you do not expect to get. If that step does not succeed, think through why not, and do whatever you can to turn disappointment into another opportunity. Many of the progressions in my own career came as a result of unexpected opportunities, following a disappointment.

Don't be afraid to take an unconventional step if there is something

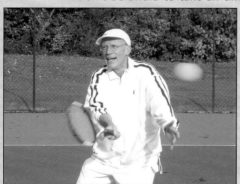

you really want to do, whether it be working abroad, doing research or taking a sideways step for a time. Whatever you are doing, do it with enthusiasm and energy, and join in and participate in as many aspects as you can.

Most of us need new challenges throughout our careers in order to maintain interest and stimulation, and there are many ways to seek them. Continuing research and other academic activities; developing a new clinical service; taking on management responsibilities; becoming involved in Royal College or other national and international organizations: these are just some of the things that invigorate and nourish our professional lives.

My own career seems to have fallen into seven-year cycles, usually when external circumstances necessitated change and thus opened other opportunities. The closure of a secondary hospital freed some time that I used in the development of an Assisted Conception Unit. The resignation of a colleague meant I had to take on administrative leadership just when the concept of clinical directors was coming in. The reorganization of hospitals into trusts created the role of medical director, allowing me to shift direction again. Later the merging of two trusts resulted in such fragmentation of clinical responsibilities that a change of consultant job was the only option. Applying for and being appointed to a new post at the age of 56 was another rejuvenating experience.

Those of us who have chosen a clinical specialty have the daily opportunity to meet and get to know a wonderfully rich and varied group of patients, from whom we can learn much. If the NHS has at times seemed frustrating, spending part of one's working week in private practice provides a refreshing change, with its greater independence and direct accountability.

Remember that arrogance, selfishness and vaulting ambition are unattractive traits; retaining a degree of modesty (as well as a sense of humour) will encourage a harmonious relationship with colleagues, patients and managers. If you can balance a satisfying and contributory professional life with a happy domestic life, allowing time for family, friends and other interests, you will have achieved success.

Professor DBA Silk MD FRCP

Consultant Physician

Ideally success should be a measure of achievement. As a cofounder of the British Association of Parenteral and Enteral Nutrition (BAPEN) in 1992, I have sought to increase the awareness and improve the management of disease-related malnutrition. Progress has been made; the increasing profile of hospital food and the recognition by politicians and the media of the importance of malnutrition is pleasing.

Many have said that if you are to succeed as a hospital doctor you must choose a specialty that interests you and that you enjoy. To this I would add that you should have received a first-class training. I was fortunate to have chosen gastroenterology as a specialty in its formative years and to have received my training in the department of Gastroenterology at St Bartholomew's Hospital and later in the Liver Unit at King's College Hospital. We were encouraged to pursue research as well as clinical medicine, a philosophy that I have continued throughout my medical career. Despite the difficulties in achieving this in the modern NHS, it is something I continue to encourage those starting out to do.

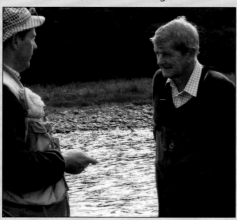

I hope that, as the picture shows, I am still not too proud to learn myself.

To the question 'Would you have changed anything in your career if you were to start out again?' I would say, firmly, no. I treasure the 26 years that I co-directed Sir Francis Avery-Jones's old unit at Central Middlesex Hospital. On the basis of our experiences, I continue to advise young gastroenterologists to learn to learn to establish relationships with their surgical colleagues and adopt a multidisciplinary approach to patient care. This has stood us in good stead in all fields of gastroenterology, particularly in the difficult functional gastrointestinal disorders and neuromuscular disorders of the gut.

Nutritional care should continue to be a link in the chain of therapy for any medical or surgical condition, and I still hope that before I retire every hospital in the country will have a well-co-ordinated multidisciplinary nutrition support team. BAPEN thinks they should, NICE thinks they should. If this comes to pass I hope some will think I have been successful as a hospital doctor.

Professor Stuart L Stanton FRCS FRCOG FRANZCOG (Hon)

Parkside Hospital, the Portland Hospital for Women & Children
and the Lister Hospital, London

I don't think I have been successful – especially when I look at the achievements of my colleagues. However, I can list the ingredients which I believe were important in my career.

- Enthusiasm – you and your team must have and show enthusiasm.
- Hard work – medicine, like many vocations, does not respect the artificial hours of 9–5, but rather you work until the job is finished.
- Humour and enjoyment – work is dull without humour, and to do a job well you must enjoy it.
- Luck and serendipity – these are often not of your making, but it helps if you are in the right place at the right time with your eyes open.
- Vision – it helps to have an aim, a vision of what you want to do and can realistically achieve.
- Role models – mine were:
    - my parents; my father introduced me to medicine and has always served as my inspiration, and my mother's approval or disapproval moved me most
    - my teachers; David Innes-Williams taught me humility and clinical competence, and 'Bodger' Chamberlain gave me encouragement as a junior and taught me team play.
- Instinct – follow your instincts and sometimes let your heart lead your head, and take a bold chance.
- Perhaps of equal importance to any of these precepts – have interests outside medicine to balance your life, chief of which should be your family, then good reading, music and sport.

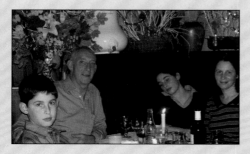

Success in medicine: voices of experience

David Weatherall FRS

Regius Professor of Medicine Emeritus, University of Oxford;
Weatherall Institute of Molecular Medicine, John Radcliffe Hospital, Oxford;
Chancellor, University of Keele

The several definitions of 'success' in the Concise Oxford Dictionary include 'the attainment of wealth, fame, or position'. Medically, this might encompass strings of degrees, a Harley Street address, a university professorship, high office in the establishment, titles and, to crown it all, a lengthy obituary in *The Times* (ideally appearing in error before one's demise).

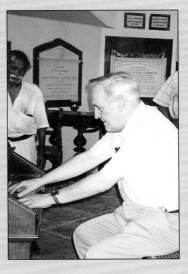

But can these accolades be equated with genuine success? Or do they just happen to some individuals by dint of hard work, ability or driving ambition, and, above all, good luck? Certainly, they do not come to equally deserving people or necessarily bring with them the satisfaction of being your own man or woman. They do not provide a sense of being at ease with yourself, or the genuine fulfilment of having done at least one thing to the very best of your ability, or even just a little better.

Is it ever possible to achieve these infinitely more worthwhile facets of success? Mentors are useful, if for nothing else than as living evidence of mistakes not to be made. Here are a few suggestions. First, do not plan your life or career in obsessive detail; those who do rarely achieve self-fulfilment or happiness. Take plenty of time to learn the basic clinical and communication skills or, if you have the burning curiosity necessary to follow a research career, the essential tools of the trade. Have a long look, both at home and abroad, at the many faces of our wonderful profession before deciding in which direction to proceed, and who to travel with. To achieve the satisfaction of doing at least one thing really well, focus on something really absorbing in a continuously self-critical way, but try to retain a broad view across medicine and the humanities. Ignore those who say there is only one pathway to career development; take some risks and be your own person from the beginning.

Remember that, although medicine is a noble profession, there is no intrinsic difference between an effective doctor and an able high-court judge or thorough roadsweeper. That occupational hazard, pomposity, is a danger to patients and precludes any possibility of coming to terms with yourself, warts and all. Humility and an ability to listen sympathetically to your patients are still the most important attributes of a successful doctor.

Pace your life and learn to say 'no'; a mind refreshed by something other than medicine or turgid administration is much more effective in the clinic or research laboratory. Later, treat young people with respect and understanding, however stupid and impossible they may seem; with increasing age, the pleasure that you will gain from their success will go some way to balancing your inevitable failures. Finally, find a partner who is sympathetic to the many trials and few successes of what, if you follow this advice, will not always be an easy ride.

Success in medicine: voices of experience

useful addresses

Action Research
Vincent House, Horsham
West Sussex RH12 2DP
Tel: 01403 210406
Fax: 01403 210541
E-mail: info@actionresearch.co.uk
http://www.actionresearch.co.uk/

Arthritis Research Campaign
Copeman House, St Mary's Court
St Mary's Gate, Chesterfield
Derbyshire S41 7TD
Tel: 01246 558033
Fax: 01246 558007
E-mail: info@arc.org.uk
http://www.arc.org.uk/

Association of Medical Research Charities
61 Gray's Inn Road, London WC1X 8TL
Tel: 020 7269 8820
Fax: 020 7269 8821
http://www.amrc.org.uk/

Association for the Study of Medical Education (ASME)
12 Queen Street, Edinburgh EH2 1JE
Tel: 0131 225 9111
Fax: 0131 225 9444
E-mail: info@asme.org.uk
http://www.asme.org.uk/

Biotechnology and Biological Sciences Research Council
Polaris House, North Star Avenue
Swindon, Wilts SN2 1UH
Tel: 01793 413200
Fax: 01793 413201
http://www.bbsrc.ac.uk/

Brain Research Trust
15 Southampton Place
London WC1A 2AJ
Tel: 020 7404 9982
Fax: 020 7404 9983
E-mail: info@brt.org.uk
http://www.brt.org.uk/

Breakthrough Breast Cancer
246 High Holborn, London WC1V 7EX
Tel: 020 7025 2400
Fax: 020 7025 2401
E-mail: info@breakthrough.org.uk
http://www.breakthrough.org.uk/

British Association of Paediatric Surgeons
Royal College of Surgeons of England
35–43 Lincoln's Inn Fields
London WC2A 3PE
Tel: 020 7869 6915
Fax: 020 7869 6919
E-mail: adminsec@baps.org.uk
http://www.baps.org.uk/

British Cardiovascular Society
9 Fitzroy Square, London W1T 5HW
Tel: 020 7383 3887
Fax: 020 7388 0903
E-mail: enquiries@bcs.com
http://www.bcs.com/

British Heart Foundation
14 Fitzhardinge Street
London W1H 6DH
Tel: 020 7935 0185
Fax: 020 7486 5820
http://www.bhf.org.uk/

British Medical Association
BMA House, Tavistock Square
London WC1H 9JP
Tel: 020 7387 4499
askBMA (BMA members only):
0870 60 60 828
Fax: 020 7383 6400
http://www.bma.org.uk/

14 Queen Street, Edinburgh EH2 ILL
Tel: 0131 247 3000
Fax: 0131 247 3001
E-mail: bmascotland@bma.org.uk

5th Floor, 2 Caspian Point
Caspian Way, Cardiff Bay
Cardiff CF10 4DQ
Tel: 029 2047 4646
Fax: 029 2047 4600
E-mail: bmawales@bma.org.uk

16 Cromac Place, Cromac Wood
Ormeau Road, Belfast BT7 2JB
Tel: 028 9026 9666
Fax: 028 9026 9665
E-mail: bmanorthernireland@bma.org.uk

BMA Counselling Services
Tel: 0645 200169 (BMA only)

British Orthopaedic Association
35–43 Lincoln's Inn Fields
London WC2A 3PE
Tel: 020 7405 6507
Fax: 020 7831 2676
http://www.boa.ac.uk/

British Postgraduate Medical
Federation
33 Millman Street, London WC1N 3EJ
Tel: 020 7831 6222
Fax: 020 7831 7599

British Urological Foundation
40 Pentonville Road, London N1 9HF
Tel: 020 7713 9538
Fax: 020 7278 5712
E-mail: info@buf.org.uk
http://www.buf.org.uk/

Cancer Research UK
PO Box 123, Lincoln's Inn Fields
London WC2A 3PX
Tel: 020 7242 0200
Fax: 020 7269 3100
http://www.cancerresearchuk.org/

Centre of Medical Law and Ethics
King's College London
Strand, London WC2R 2LS
Tel: 020 7848 2382
Fax: 020 7848 2575
E-mail: cmle.enq@kcl.ac.uk
http://www.kcl.ac.uk/schools/law/resea
rch/cmle/

Cystic Fibrosis Trust
11 London Road
Bromley, Kent BR1 1BY
Tel: 020 8464 7211
Fax: 020 8313 0472
enquiries@cftrust.org.uk
http://www.cftrust.org.uk/

Department of Health
Public Enquiry Office
Richmond House
79 Whitehall, London SW1A 2NS
Tel: 020 7210 4850
E-mail: dhmail@dh.gsi.gov.uk
http://www.dh.gov.uk/

Engineering and Physical Sciences
Research Council
Polaris House, North Star Avenue
Swindon, Wilts SN2 1ET
Tel: 01793 444100
E-mail: infoline@epsrc.ac.uk
http://www.epsrc.ac.uk/

European Commission
200 rue de la Loi / Wetstraat 200
B-1049 Brussels, Belgium
Tel: 00 32 2299 1111
http://ec.europa.eu/index_en.htm

Faculty of Dental Surgery
Royal College of Surgeons of England
35–43 Lincoln's Inn Fields
London WC2A 3PE
Tel: 020 7869 6810
Fax: 020 7869 6816
E-mail: fds@rcseng.ac.uk

Faculty of Occupational Medicine of
the Royal College of Physicians
6 St Andrew's Place
Regent's Park, London NW1 4LB
Tel: 020 7317 5890
Fax: 020 7317 5899
http://www.facoccmed.ac.uk/

Faculty of Public Health Medicine
4 St Andrew's Place
Regent's Park, London NW1 4LB
Tel: 020 7935 0243
Fax: 020 7224 6973
E-mail: enquiries@fphm.org.uk
http://www.fph.org.uk/

Fellowship of Postgraduate Medicine
12 Chandos Street, London W1M 9DE
Tel: 020 7636 6334
Fax: 020 7436 2535

General Dental Council
37 Wimpole Street, London W1G 8DQ
Tel: 020 7887 3800
Fax: 020 7224 3294
http://www.gdc-uk.org/

General Medical Council
Regent's Place, 350 Euston Road
London NW1 3JN
Tel: 0845 357 3456
E-mail: gmc@gmc-uk.org
http://www.gmc-uk.org/

Higher Education Funding Council
for England (HEFCE)
Northavon House, Coldharbour Lane
Bristol BS16 1QD
Tel: 0117 931 7317
Fax: 0117 931 7203
E-mail: hefce@hefce.ac.uk
http://www.hefce.ac.uk

Hospice Information
Help the Hospices
Hospice House
34–44 Britannia Street
London WC1X 9JG
Tel: 020 7520 8232
http://www.hospiceinformation.info/

Hospital Consultants and Specialists
Association
1 Kingsclere Road, Overton
Basingstoke RG25 3JA
Tel: 01256 771777
Fax: 01256 770999
E-mail: conspec@hcsa.com
http://www.hcsa.com/

Independent Doctors' Forum
http://www.independentdoctorsforum.
net/

Institute of Healthcare Management
18–21 Morley Street
London SE1 7QZ
Tel: 020 7620 1030
Fax: 020 7620 1040
E-mail: enquiries@ihm.org.uk
http://www.ihm.org.uk/

Intensive Care Society
Churchill House, 35 Red Lion Square
London WC1R 4SG
Tel: 020 7280 4350
Fax: 020 7280 4369
http://www.ics.ac.uk/

Intercollegiate Surgical Curriculum
Project
http://www.iscp.ac.uk/

Joint Committee on Higher Medical
Training
5 St Andrew's Place, Regent's Park
London NW1 4LB
Tel: 020 7935 1174
Fax: 0207 486 4160
E-mail: hmt@rcplondon.ac.uk
http://www.jchmt.org.uk/

Joint Committee on Higher
Psychiatric Training
c/o Royal College of Psychiatrists
17 Belgrave Square
London SW1X 8PG
Tel: 020 7235 2351

Joint Committee on Higher Surgical
Training
Royal Colleges of Surgeons
35–43 Lincoln's Inn Fields
London WC2A 3PE
Tel: 020 7405 3474
E-mail: jchst@jchst.org/
http://www.jchst.org/

Kidney Research UK
Kings Chambers, Priestgate
Peterborough PE1 1FG
Tel: 01733 704650 / 0845 070 7601
E-mail: communications@kidney
researchuk.org
http://www.nkrf.org.uk/

King's Fund
11–13 Cavendish Square
London W1G 0AN
Tel: 020 7307 2400
Fax: 020 7307 2801
http://www.kingsfund.org.uk/

London Consultants' Association
14 Queen Anne's Gate
London SW1H 9AA
Tel: 020 7222 0975
Fax: 020 7222 4424
http://www.london-consultants.
org.uk/

Marie Curie Research Institute
The Chart, Oxted, Surrey RH8 0TL
Tel: 01883 722306
Fax: 01883 714375
http://www.mcri.ac.uk/

Macmillan Cancer Support
89 Albert Embankment
London SE1 7UQ
http://www.macmillan.org.uk/

Medical Defence Union
230 Blackfriars Road, London SE1 8PJ
Tel: 020 7202 1500
E-mail: mdu@the-mdu.com
http://www.the-mdu.com/

**Medical Interview Teaching
Association (MITA)**
http://www.mita.soton.ac.uk/

Medical Protection Society
33 Cavendish Square
London W1G 0PS
Tel: 020 7399 1300
Fax: 020 7399 1301
E-mail: info@mps.org.uk
http://www.medicalprotection.org/

Medical Research Council
(includes National Institute for
Medical Research)
20 Park Crescent, London W1B 4AL
Tel: 020 7636 5422
Fax: 020 7436 6179
E-mail: corporate@headoffice.mrc.ac.uk
http://www.mrc.ac.uk/

Medical Women's Federation
Tavistock House North
Tavistock Square
London WC1H 9HX
Tel: 020 7387 7765
Fax: 020 7388 9216
E-mail: admin.mwf@btconnect.com
http://www.medicalwomensfederation
.org.uk/

Medicines and Healthcare products
Regulatory Agency
10-2 Market Towers, 1 Nine Elms Lane
London SW8 5NQ
Tel: 020 7084 2000 (weekdays
0900–1700)
Tel: 020 7210 3000 (other times)
Fax: 020 7084 2353
E-mail: info@mhra.gsi.gov.uk
http://www.mhra.gov.uk/

Men's Health Forum
Tavistock House, Tavistock Square
London WC1H 9HR
Tel: 020 7388 4449
Fax: 020 7388 4477
http://www.menshealthforum.org.uk/

Mental Health Foundation
9th Floor, Sea Containers House
20 Upper Ground, London SE1 9QB
Tel: 020 7580 0145
Fax: 020 7631 3868

Merchants House, 30 George Square
Glasgow G2 1EG
E-mail: mhf@mhf.org.uk
http://www.mentalhealth.org.uk/

Migraine Trust
55–56 Russell Square
London WC1B 4HP
Tel: 020 7436 1336
Fax: 020 7436 2880
E-mail: info@migrainetrust.org
http://www.migrainetrust.org/

Modernising Medical Careers
New Kings Beam House, 6th Floor
22 Upper Ground, London SE1 9PJ
http://www.mmc.nhs.uk/

Muscular Dystrophy Campaign
7–11 Prescott Place, London SW4 6BS
Tel: 020 7720 8055
Fax: 020 7498 0670
E-mail: info@muscular-dystrophy.org
www.muscular-dystrophy.org

Multiple Sclerosis Society
372 Edgware Road, London, NW2 6ND
Tel: 020 8438 0700
http://www.mssociety.org.uk/

National Advice Centre for
Postgraduate Medical Education
PO Box 2516, St James House
Bristol, BS2 2AA
Tel: 0117 915 7069
Fax: 0117 915 6721
E-mail: nacpme@nhscareers.nhs.uk
http://www.nhscareers.nhs.uk/

National Institute for Health and
Clinical Excellence
MidCity Place, 71 High Holborn
London, WC1V 6NA
Tel: 020 7067 5800
Fax: 020 7067 5801
E-mail: nice@nice.org.uk
http://www.nice.org.uk/

National Osteoporosis Society
Camerton, Bath BA2 0PJ
Tel: 01761 471771 / 0845 130 3076
Fax: 01761 471104
E-mail: info@nos.org.uk
http://www.nos.org.uk/

NHS Confederation
29 Bressenden Place
London SW1E 5DD
Tel: 020 7074 3200
Fax: 020 7074 3201
http://www.nhsconfed.org/

No Free Lunch UK
http://www.nofreelunch-uk.org/

Open University Centre for Education for Medicine
Crowther 208, Walton Hall
Milton Keynes MK7 6AA
Tel: 01908 653776
Fax: 01908 659374
E-mail: oucem@open.ac.uk
http://iet.open.ac.uk/about/oucem/

Postgraduate Medical Education and Training Board (PMETB)
7th Floor, Hercules House
London SE1 7DU
Tel: 020 7160 6100
Fax: 020 7160 6102
http://www.pmetb.org.uk/

Prostate Cancer Charity
3 Angel Walk, London W6 9HX
Tel: 020 8222 7622
Fax: 020 8222 7639
E-mail: info@prostate-cancer.org.uk
http://www.prostate-cancer.org.uk/

Prostate Research Campaign UK
10 Northfields Prospect
Putney Bridge Road
London SW18 1PE
Tel: 020 8877 5840
Fax: 020 8877 2609
E-mail: info@prostate-research.org.uk
http://www.prostate-research.org.uk/

Research into Ageing
Help the Aged
207–221 Pentonville Road
London N1 9UZ
Tel: 020 7278 1114
Fax: 020 7278 1116
E-mail: info@helptheaged.org.uk
http://www.ageing.org/

Royal College of Anaesthetists
Churchill House, 35 Red Lion Square
London WC1R 4SG
Tel: 020 7092 1500
Fax: 020 7092 1730
E-mail: info@rcoa.ac.uk
http://www.rcoa.ac.uk/

Royal College of General
Practitioners
14 Princes Gate, Hyde Park
London SW7 1PU
Tel: 020 7581 3232 / 0845 456 4041
Fax: 020 7225 3047
E-mail: info@rcgp.org.uk
http://www.rcgp.org.uk/

Royal College of Obstetricians and
Gynaecologists
27 Sussex Place, Regent's Park
London NW1 4RG
Tel: 020 7772 6220
Fax: 020 7723 0575
http://www.rcog.org.uk/

Royal College of Ophthalmologists
17 Cornwall Terrace, London NW1 4QW
Tel: 020 7935 0702
Fax: 020 7935 9838
http://www.rcophth.ac.uk/

Royal College of Paediatrics and
Child Health
50 Hallam Street, London W1W 6DE
Tel: 020 7307 5600
Fax: 020 7307 5601
E-mail: enquiries@rcpch.ac.uk
http://www.rcpch.ac.uk/

Royal College of Pathologists
2 Carlton House Terrace
London SW1Y 5AF
Tel: 020 7451 6700
Fax: 020 7451 6701
E-mail: info@rcpath.org
http://www.rcpath.org/

Royal College of Physicians of
Edinburgh
9 Queen Street, Edinburgh EH2 1JQ
Tel: 0131 225 7324
Fax: 0131 220 3939
http://www.rcpe.ac.uk/

Royal College of Physicians of
London
11 St Andrew's Place, Regent's Park
London NW1 4LE
Tel: 020 7935 1174
Fax: 020 7487 5218
http://www.rcplondon.ac.uk/

Royal College of Physicians and
Surgeons of Glasgow
232–234 St Vincent Street
Glasgow G2 5RJ
Tel: 0141 221 6072
Fax: 0141 221 1804
http://www.rcpsg.ac.uk/

Royal College of Psychiatrists
17 Belgrave Square
London SW1X 8PG
Tel: 020 7235 2351
Fax: 020 7245 1231
E-mail: rcpsych@rcpsych.ac.uk
http://www.rcpsych.ac.uk/

Royal College of Radiologists
38 Portland Place, London W1B 1JQ
Tel: 020 7636 4432
Fax: 020 7323 3100
E-mail: enquiries@rcr.ac.uk
http://www.rcr.ac.uk/

Royal College of Surgeons of
Edinburgh
Nicolson Street, Edinburgh EH8 9DW
Tel: 0131 527 1600
Fax: 0131 557 6406
E-mail: information@rcsed.ac.uk
http://www.rcsed.ac.uk/

Royal College of Surgeons of
England
35–43 Lincoln's Inn Fields
London WC2A 3PE
Tel: 020 7405 3474
Fax: 020 7973 2135
http://www.rcseng.ac.uk/

Royal Medical Society
Student Centre, 5/5 Bristo Square
Edinburgh EH8 9AL
Tel: 0131 650 2672
E-mail: enquiries@royalmedical.co.uk
http://www.royalmedicalsociety.co.uk/

Royal Society for the Promotion
of Health
RSH House, 38A St George's Drive
London SW1V 4BH
Tel: 020 7630 0121
Fax: 020 7976 6847
E-mail: rsph@rsph.org
http://www.rsph.org/

Royal Society of Medicine
1 Wimpole Street, London W1G 0AE
Tel: 020 7290 2900
Fax: 020 7290 2909
http://www.roysocmed.ac.uk/

Smith and Nephew Foundation
15 Adam Street, London WC2N 6LA
Tel: 020 7960 2276
E-mail: foundation.enquiries@smith-
nephew.com
http://www.snfoundation.org.uk/

Wellbeing of Women
27 Sussex Place, Regent's Park
London NW1 4SP
Tel: 020 7772 6400
Fax: 020 7724 7725
http://www.wellbeingofwomen.org.uk/

Wellcome Trust
215 Euston Road, London NW1 2BE
Tel: 020 7611 8888
Fax: 020 7611 8545
E-mail: contact@wellcome.ac.uk
http://www.wellcome.ac.uk/

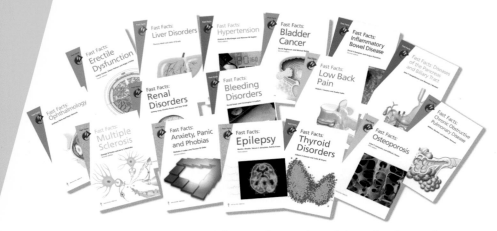